supplied by:-
RADIO SCHOOL
33 Island Close
HAYLING ISLAND
Hants. PO11 0NJ
Tel: (0705) 466450

MARINE VHF OPERATION

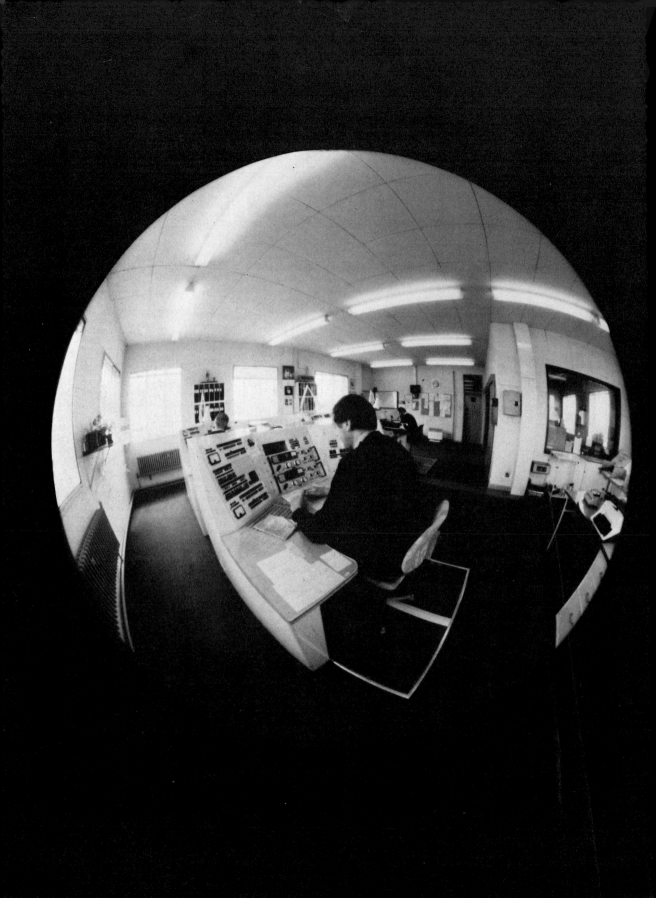

MARINE VHF OPERATION

J. Michael Gale

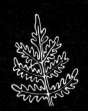

Fernhurst Books

First published 1987 by
Fernhurst Books, 31 Church Road, Hove, East Sussex

ISBN 0 906754 27 5

Phototypesetting: Foxash Typesetters, Steyning
Artwork: PanTek, Maidstone
Printed by Ebenezer Baylis & Son Ltd, Worcester

Acknowledgements
The author and publishers would like to thank Mike Peyton for drawing the cartoons, and ICOM (UK) Ltd (sole importers of ICOM radio communications equipment) for their assistance in the preparation of the book and for supplying the photographs credited below. Thanks are also due to Kelvin Hughes Ltd for their advice on the manuscript.

Photo credits
BTI Maritime Radio: pages 2, 21
Department of Trade and Industry: pages 9, 44
J. Michael Gale: pages 16, 17 18
Tim Hore: pages 12, 37
ICOM (UK) Ltd: front cover, 25

Preceding page: The main operating room of a Coast Radio Station.

Contents

1 Certificates and licences

Having acquired a marine radiotelephone you have to licence it. The documents required are very similar to those needed for a car.

Operator's certificate

Just as every driver must have passed a Driving Test to qualify for a Driving Licence, so a marine radiotelephone set must be *controlled* by an authorised operator who has passed an examination to qualify for a Certificate of Competence in Radiotelephony, and who has been granted an Authority to Operate in British Ships. Examinations for the 'VHF Only' certificate are conducted by the Royal Yachting Association (RYA) at a number of nautical colleges and local colleges of education throughout Britain. The RYA also hold 'VHF Only' examinations at important Boat Shows for which prior application *must* be made to the RYA. Addresses of examination centres are listed at the back of this book, together with that of the RYA which can supply the dates of examinations.

Anyone on board may *use* the radiotelephone provided it is *controlled* by an Authorised Operator (Q15). Anyone of any age or nationality may be awarded the Certificate of Competence upon successful examination but you must be at least 16 years old to be granted the Authority to Operate. The Certificate of Competence and Authority to Operate last for the life of the holder and do not have to be renewed.

The examination

The 'VHF only' examination takes about an hour and consists of a fifteen-question written paper, for which 30 minutes is allowed, followed by a few oral questions and a practical test on a VHF simulator. The full syllabus and 'question bank', from which several exam papers have compiled, is contained in RYA booklet G26.

In these pages, the author has answered most of the questions likely to be found in the half-hour written paper. Throughout the text, every statement which answers one of these examination questions is followed by the question number in brackets.

Having passed the examination, the holder is qualified to operate the VHF radiotelephone in any British ship in any part of the world for the rest of the holder's life. But *only* the 25 watt (Q7) short-range VHF R/T. To operate the 400 watt medium-range MF (Medium Wave) and 1500 watt long-range HF (Short Wave) Single-Sideband equipment, a higher grade certificate such as the 'Restricted' certificate is required.

Ship's licence

Just as a Vehicle Licence is required if a car is to be used on a public road, so a DTI Ship Radio Licence is required if a radiotelephone is to be installed and used in a vessel (Q15). The dealer who supplied the set should be able to supply the application form but, if not, it can be obtained from the Department of Trade & Industry (see list of addresses at the back of this book).

Like the Vehicle Licence, the Ship Radio Licence is renewable annually. New VHF installations are not inspected as a matter of routine but random spot checks are made periodically by the Radio Investigation Service of the DTI. They have powers of immediate confiscation of unlicensed equipment and prosecution of the owner. The Ship's Radio Licence, Operator's Certificate and a copy of Section 11 of the Post Office (Protection) Act 1884 (supplied with the Ship's Licence) *must be kept on board* for inspection by an authorised officer of any government.

Most of the application form for the Ship Radio Licence is self-explanatory but some sections require some clarification.

Para. 4 'Call-sign'

When a vessel is first licensed for radio (the *vessel* is licensed, not the set) it is allocated a call-sign by the DTI in exactly the same way that a vehicle is

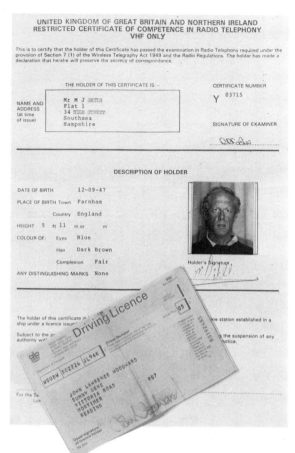

Above: The radio operator's licence corresponds to the licence held by every qualified driver.

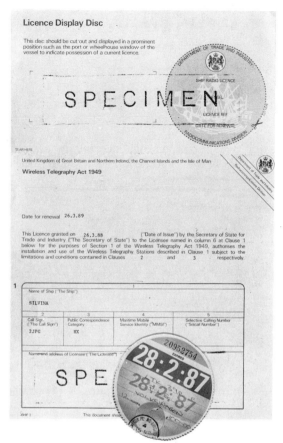

Above: The ship's licence corresponds to the tax disc displayed on every vehicle used on the road.

allocated a registration number when it is first licensed for the road. Once allocated, the call-sign remains with the vessel irrespective of change of ownership, change of vessel name or whether the licence is renewed, so long as the vessel remains in British hands.

As well as providing a unique identification, the first digit (or two) indicates the station's nationality (Q10). The first digit of all British radio stations (land, ship or aircraft) is a 'G' or 'M' or '2'. For example, the author's Amateur Radio call-sign is G3JMG and a yacht once owned is 2JPG (spoken as 'Two Juliet Papa Golf'). A typical present-day yacht's call-sign would be MXYZ6 (spoken as 'Mike X-ray Yankee Zulu Six').

If your vessel is new or has never been fitted with radio, leave paragraph 4 blank or write 'new vessel' and a call-sign will be allocated. If your vessel already has a call-sign, enter it paragraph 4. If your vessel has a radio, or you think it may have

had in the past, try to discover the call-sign from the previous owner(s). If a call-sign cannot be traced, complete paragraphs 5 and 6.

Para. 13 'Will communication with foreign Coast Stations be required?'

With your VHF R/T you may talk directly and at no charge to coastguards, VHF-equipped vessels, harbourmasters, marinas and yacht clubs. You can also be connected to the world's telephone system for making telephone calls to or from the shore, via a world-wide network of shore-side radio 'telephone exchanges' called Coast Radio Stations. Unfortunately telephone calls must be paid for! As a coin-box cannot be fitted to your VHF set, an account must be opened with an Authorised Radio Company for calls via foreign Coast Radio Stations. British yacht owners are advised to appoint British Telecom by entering 'GB14' in paragraph 13.

2 The phonetic alphabet

For accuracy in communication, it is absolutely vital that every radio or telephone operator is fluent in the phonetic alphabet. When talking over the radio or telephone, it can be almost impossible to distinguish between 'F' and 'S', 'N' and 'M', or 'B' and 'P'. To ensure accuracy, a name or uncommon word may be spelled out using a word for each letter.

This technique originated in the First World War with the 'ACK-ACK, BEER-BEER' system. Veterans may remember the example used to illustrate the necessity of such a system when a message reputedly started out in a trench as 'Send reinforcements, we are going to advance' but ended up at Battalion HQ as 'Send three and fourpence, we are going to a dance'! Certainly some years ago, a student telephoned the author to ask exactly where, in Salisbury, a class was being held. When asked why he thought it was being held in Salisbury, he replied 'Your wife told me the address was Wickham Road, Sarum' (Sarum is the old name for Salisbury). To which the reply was 'No she didn't – she said Wickham Road, *Fareham*. I SPELL "FOXTROT, ALPHA, ROMEO, ECHO, HOTEL, ALPHA, MIKE" '.

The example quoted uses the current system, introduced on 1st January 1955 for NATO forces and replacing the Second World War system. Originally used for military purposes only, it became so successful that it is now used for *all* marine and aeronautical radio throughout the world (Q8). Note that when spelling out a word phonetically, it is essential to say 'I SPELL' before launching into phonetics; this is a signal for the recipient to put pencil to paper and take down the message.

Phonetic alphabet

Letter	Word	Spoken as	Variations	Letter	Word	Spoken as	
A	ALPHA	AL-fah		K	KILO	KEE-loh	
B	BRAVO	BRA-voh		L	LIMA	LEE-mah	
C	CHARLIE	CHAR-lee	French may say 'SHAR-lee'	M	MIKE	MIKE	
				N	NOVEMBER	no-VEM-bah	
				O	OSCAR	OSS-kar	
				P	PAPA	pa-PAH	
				Q	QUEBEC	key-BECK	
D	DELTA	DELL-tah		R	ROMEO	ROW-mee-oh	
E	ECHO	ECK-oh		S	SIERRA	see-AIR-rah	
F	FOXTROT	FOKS-trot		T	TANGO	TANG-go	
G	GOLF	GOLF		U	UNIFORM	YOU-nee-form	
H	HOTEL	hoh-TELL	French may say 'oh-TELL'	V	VICTOR	VIK-tah	
				W	WHISKEY	WISS-key	Germans may say 'VISS-key'.
I	INDIA	IN-dee-ah					
J	JULIETT	JEW-lee-ETT	Germans may say 'YOU-lee-ett'	X	X-RAY	ECKS-ray	
				Y	YANKEE	YANG-key	
				Z	ZULU	ZOO-loo	

Phonetic numerals

There is also a system of International phonetic numerals but it is rarely used as most communicators throughout the world say numerals in English. However, there is still some possibility of confusion, particularly with 'five' and 'nine', so it is usual to shorten 'five' to 'FIFE' and extend 'nine' into 'NINER' to help distinguish between them. Here is the complete list:

Numeral	Spoken as
1	WUN
2	TOO
3	TREE
4	FOW-er
5	FIFE
6	SIX
7	SEV-en
8	AIT
9	NINE-er
0	ZERO

Do not say 'OH' for '0' as it can sound like 'TWO'. Numbers should be spoken figure-by-figure except for whole thousands, and if a decimal point occurs in a number, it is given as 'point'. For example:

Numeral	Spoken as
32	TREE TOO
459	FOW-er, FIFE, NINE-er
200	TOO, ZERO, ZERO
8162	AIT, WUN, SIX, TOO
7000	SEV-en TOUSAND
2.5	TOO POINT FIFE

Below: Spelling out the ship's name and call-sign in phonetics not only ensures accuracy; it also gives the radio operator at the other end the opportunity to write down each letter in sequence.

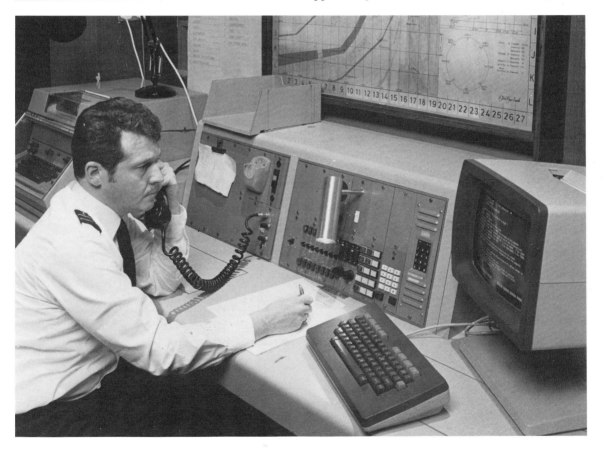

3 Organisation of the marine VHF band

To use your VHF set to full advantage (and pass the exam) it is essential to have a thorough understanding of the organisation of the marine VHF band which is quite different from any other radio band.

Radio 'frequency' means 'cycles-per-second'. A frequency of one cycle per second is expressed as one Hertz (1 Hz), after the German physicist and radio pioneer H. R. Hertz. For convenience, the whole range of radio frequencies is divided into a number of groups or 'bands' according to frequency range. Marine VHF operation is carried out within the Very High Frequency (VHF) band which ranges from 30 megahertz (MHz) to 300 MHz, that is 30-300 million cycles per second (between ten metres and one metre wavelength). If you have a VHF band on your domestic radio (it may be marked 'FM' or, if of German make, 'UKW') you will see that the dial is marked from 88 to 108. These are the limits, in MHz, of the *broadcasting* part of the VHF band – around three metres in wavelength.

International channels

The limits of what is called the International Maritime Mobile (IMM) Band are 156 MHz to 162 MHz. So, although we are operating in the same VHF band as the BBC, we are operating in a different part of it, which is why we do not hear the BBC on our marine VHF R/T – or ships on our domestic radio.

Between the limits of 156-162 MHz, the IMM Band is further sub-divided into a number of small segments or 'channels'. Each channel is numbered for convenience, because we are dealing in hundreds of megahertz to two or three decimal places, which even professionals have difficulty in remembering. The use of numbered channels makes for very easy operation of the set; simply turn the knob (or push the button) for the appropriate channel number. The actual frequencies involved are of purely academic interest.

The channelling of the IMM Band was re-arranged on 1st January 1972 which makes the present scheme look highly complex and very illogical. To make for easier understanding, consider first the original scheme which was introduced soon after the Second World War. As you see from Table 1, the channels were numbered consecutively from 1 to 28 (although there is a Channel 00 on 156.000 MHz, it is for HM Coastguards' own private use). In this respect, the IMM Band is like the present Citizen's Band (CB) which is similarly divided into 40 numbered channels. However, the big difference lies in the fact that whereas every CB operator is fully authorised to use *any* of his 40 channels for any purpose, the marine VHF operator has to choose a channel which is appropriate for the use intended. As you see from Table 1, every channel in the IMM Band is dedicated to a particular use. Some channels are dedicated exclusively but others are shared (Q5).

In ship-to-shore communication, the shore station dictates the particular channel but with inter-ship communication, it is the *station called* which nominates the channel (Q11). Thus *it is only with inter-ship operation that the on-ship operator ever gets the chance to nominate a channel.*

Channel 16
From Table 1, you can see that Channels 06, 08, 09, 10, 13, 15 or 17 can be used for talking to friends on other boats – but how do you know which channel your friends are listening on? The answer is that you wouldn't know, were it not that one channel, Channel 16, has been set aside for CALLING. It is also used for Distress and Urgency messages. Hence it is important to keep any operation on Channel 16 to a minimum.

Channel 16 acts as a central 'meeting place' or 'clearing house' where everybody first meets everybody else before changing to an appropriate working channel, as the others are called. The usual procedure for vessels, therefore, is to leave the set switched on and listening to Ch. 16 all the time you are on board. If anyone wants to talk to you *they will first call on Ch. 16*. Also, should a sudden emergency arise, Ch. 16 is the one on

TABLE 1: INTERNATIONAL CHANNELS (BASIC)

Channel no.	Ship station frequency	Shore station frequency	Function of channel
00	156.000	156.000	H.M. COASTGUARD – PRIVATE
01	156.050	160.650	PUBLIC CORRESPONDENCE & PORT OPERATIONS (TWO FREQUENCY)
02	156.100	160.700	
03	156.150	160.750	
04	156.200	160.800	
05	156.250	160.850	
06	156.300	—	INTER-SHIP *ONLY*
07	156.350	160.950	PUBLIC CORR. & PORT OPS
08	156.400	—	INTER-SHIP *ONLY*
09	156.450	156.450	INTER-SHIP & PORT OPERATIONS
10	156.500	156.500	
11	156.550	156.550	PORT OPERATIONS *ONLY*
12	156.600	156.600	
13	156.650	156.650	INTER-SHIP & PORT OPERATIONS
14	156.700	156.700	PORT OPERATIONS *ONLY*
15	156.750	156.750	INTER-SHIP & PORT OPERATIONS
16	156.800	156.800	DISTRESS, URGENCY & CALLING *ONLY*
17	156.850	156.850	INTER-SHIP & PORT OPERATIONS
18	156.900	161.500	PORT OPERATIONS *ONLY* (TWO-FREQUENCY)
19	156.950	161.550	
20	157.000	161.600	
21	157.050	161.650	
22	157.100	161.700	
23	157.150	161.750	PUBLIC CORRESPONDENCE *ONLY* (TWO-FREQUENCY)
24	157.200	161.800	
25	157.250	161.850	
26	157.300	161.900	
27	157.350	161.950	
28	157.400	162.000	

which the distress or urgency message will be sent.

Although this is the *usual* procedure, there are now an increasing number of exceptions and alternatives to the general rule of making the initial call on Ch. 16. The precise procedure for calling specific radio stations is given in chapters 7-12 below.

Two-frequency channels

Look closely at the frequencies allocated to each channel (Table 1) and you will notice that the channels in the centre of the band between Ch. 8 and Ch. 17, for Inter-ship and Port Operations use, have been allocated a single frequency for both ship and shore stations. For example, if you call a harbourmaster on Ch. 16 and he says 'go to Ch. 12' both you and he switch to Channel 12 and speak to each other on 156.6 MHz. In other words you are both talking, literally, 'on the same wavelength'.

However, channels at the low-frequency and high-frequency end of the band (1-5, 7 and 18-28) which are used principally for 'Public Correspondence' (telephone calls to the shore) have been allocated *two* frequencies: one for the ship and a completely different one for the shore station. For example, if you call Niton Radio for a telephone call on Ch. 04 (Coast Radio Stations are called directly on one of the working channels, not Ch. 16 – see chapter 10) your transmission is made on 156.2 MHz. Niton Radio must therefore listen for you on 156.2 MHz, which he does, so he hears you. However, his transmission is made on 160.8 MHz – a completely different frequency. To receive his

transmission, therefore, your *receiver* must be tuned to 160.8 MHz – which it is, so you hear him. In practice there is no need to worry about this when making such a call, as the separate transmit and receive frequencies are automatically sorted out within your set when you select the appropriate channel number.

It is essential that you are aware that this situation exists, though, because on the two-frequency channels you can talk *only* to the appropriate shore station; it is *technically impossible* to talk to other vessels. This confuses unqualified operators who mistakenly believe that the marine VHF band operates as a sort of 'maritime CB' which merely involves selecting a channel which no-one else is using. If the chosen channel is a two-frequency one, they will be disappointed. For example: in British waters you will rarely hear anything on Ch. 03; few British

Below: Use the exclusive inter-ship channels 06, 08, 72 and 77 when speaking to other vessels.

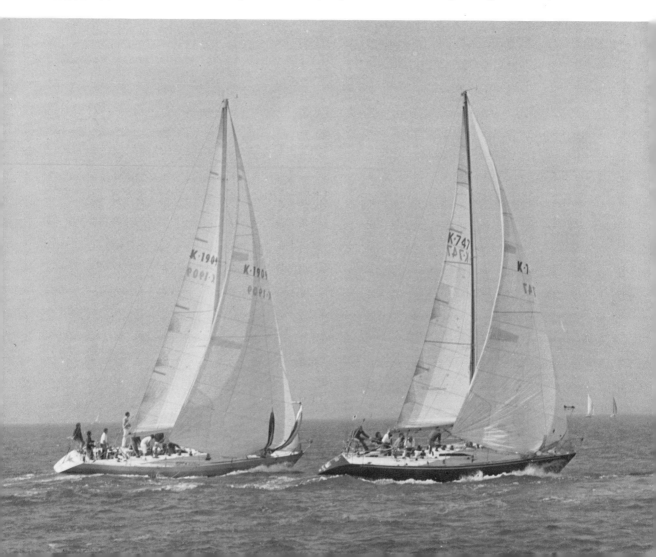

shore stations use this channel so it always seems to be available for use. It is *not*, because it is a two-frequency channel. So if you hear a vessel call another on Ch. 16 and suggest switching to Ch. 03, you know that they are unqualified. One station will make a transmission on 156.15 MHz but the other will be listening on 160.75 MHz. They will *never* hear each other! (Q14).

You can talk to the appropriate shore station on a two-frequency channel because their transmitting and receiving frequencies are the opposite to yours: they are listening on your transmitting frequency and transmitting on your listening frequency. But every other vessel is the *same* as yours. On Ch. 03, for example, all vessels transmit on 156.15 MHz but listen on 160.75 MHz. *This cannot be altered.*

Channels to avoid

Although it is technically possible to talk to another vessel on any single-frequency channel, there are a number which should not be used. Ch. 11, 12, and 14 are reserved *exclusively* for harbour authorities. Other channels, although theoretically available for inter-ship communication, should also be avoided. Do not use Ch. 13 in the Portsmouth, Weymouth, Plymouth and Clyde areas as the Queens' Harbourmaster at all British naval bases uses this channel for talking to warships. Similarly, avoid Ch. 09 inter-ship, especially in the vicinity of major ports, as it is used by UK pilot vessels and harbour tugs. In the UK, Ch. 10 is used for pollution control activities.

In general, it is best to stick to the exclusive inter-ship channels of which there are now four: 06, 08, 72 and 77.

Interleaved channels

By the early 1970s, the great increase in the use of marine VHF was causing congestion on the 28 channels available. More channels were needed but the IMM Band limits could not be extended. Instead, the width of each channel was reduced.

Reference to Table 1 shows that the channels were originally 50 kHz wide and were spaced at 50 kHz intervals. For example: Ch. 01 is centred on 156.05 MHz and Ch. 02 on 156.1, which is 50 kHz higher. On 1st January 1972, the width of all marine VHF channels was decreased from their original 50 kHz to the present 25 kHz. Thus a gap, also 25 kHz wide, appeared between each of the original channels. In this way, the number of channels was doubled overnight without extending the limits and all marine VHF equipment was altered to suit. However, this caused a small problem with the numbering system. Rather than scrap the original system and start afresh by renumbering the channels 1-56, the original numbers were retained on the original channels. The interleaved channels, as they are known, were given completely fresh numbers. Unfortunately, numbers 29-59 had already been allocated to other services so the first number available was 60. This gave rise to the rather odd present situation seen in Table 2. This confuses the uninitiated who buy what is advertised as a 55 channel marine VHF set and are delighted to find that it actually goes up to Ch. 88. Their initial delight turns to dismay when they find that Channels 29 to 59 seem to be missing!

Private channels

Look closely at Table 2 and you will see that a large number of *frequencies* are missing. The highest transmitting frequency (Ch. 88) is 157.425 MHz but the lowest receiving frequency in column 3 (Ch. 60) is 160.625 MHz.

These 'missing' frequencies are also divided into channels for *private* use. Every qualified marine radiotelephone operator is fully authorised to use any of the international channels in Table 2 but, in addition, every maritime government may authorise its nationals to operate on one or more of these 'missing' frequencies on a private and exclusive basis. These private channels, as they are known, are allocated to corporate bodies such as ferry companies, towing and salvage companies.

The British Government has allocated two of the private channels for the use of British yacht clubs. The first, on 157.85 MHz and called Channel 'M', is also shared with British marinas. If your set cannot display 'M', you may have to select '37' or 'P1' or press a dedicated button. In 1989, a second private channel on 161.425 MHz, called 'M2', was released for British yacht clubs *only* together with International Channel 80 for British marinas *only*. It should be noted that, with one exception, British yacht clubs and marinas are not licensed for Ch. 16 and must, therefore, be *called directly* on the working channel.

As a point of interest, the private channels also occupy the range of frequencies from 162.05 MHz to 174.00 MHz.

TABLE 2: INTERNATIONAL CHANNELS (INTERLEAVED)			
Channel no.		**Ship station frequency**	**Shore station frequency**	**Function of channel**

Channel no.		Ship station frequency	Shore station frequency	Function of channel
00		156.000	156.000	H.M. COASTGUARD – PRIVATE
	60	156.025	160.625	PUBLIC CORRESPONDENCE & PORT OPERATIONS (TWO-FREQUENCY)
01		156.050	160.650	
	61	156.075	160.675	
02		156.100	160.700	
	62	156.125	160.725	
03		156.150	160.750	
	63	156.175	160.775	
04		156.200	160.800	
	64	156.225	160.825	
05		156.250	160.850	
	65	156.275	160.875	
06		156.300	—	INTER-SHIP *ONLY*
	66	156.325	160.925	PUBLIC CORRESPONDENCE & PORT OPERATIONS
07		156.350	160.950	
	67	156.375	156.375	HMCG PRIMARY SAFETY CHANNEL
08		156.400	—	INTER-SHIP *ONLY*
	68	156.425	156.425	PORT OPERATIONS *ONLY*
09		156.450	156.450	INTER-SHIP & PORT OPERATIONS (Ch. 10 UK POLLUTION CONTROL)
	69	156.475	156.475	
10		156.500	156.500	
	70	156.525	DIGITAL	SELECTIVE CALL-DISTRESS & SAFETY
11		156.550	156.550	PORT OPERATIONS *ONLY*
	71	156.575	156.575	
12		156.600	156.600	
	72	156.625	—	INTER-SHIP *ONLY*
13		156.650	156.650	INTER-SHIP & PORT OPERATIONS (Ch. 73 UK SECONDARY SAFETY CHANNEL)
	73	156.675	156.675	
14		156.700	156.700	PORT OPERATIONS *ONLY*
	74	156.725	156.725	

Channel no.		Ship station frequency	Shore station frequency	Function of channel
15		156.750	156.750	INTER-SHIP & PORT OPERATIONS
	75	—	—	GUARD BAND 156.7625 – 156.7875 MHz
16		156.800	156.800	DISTRESS, URGENCY & CALLING *ONLY*
	76	156.825	156.825	DIRECT-PRINTING TELEGRAPHY FOR DISTRESS & SAFETY
17		156.850	156.850	INTER-SHIP & PORT OPERATIONS
	77	156.875	—	INTER-SHIP *ONLY*
18		156.900	161.500	PORT OPERATIONS *ONLY*
	78	156.925	161.525	PUBLIC CORR. & PORT OPERATIONS
19		156.950	161.550	PORT OPERATIONS *ONLY* (TWO-FREQUENCY)
	79	156.975	161.575	
20		157.000	161.600	
	80	157.025	161.625	
21		157.050	161.650	
	81	157.075	161.675	PUBLIC CORR. & PORT OPERATIONS
22		157.100	161.700	PORT OPERATIONS *ONLY*
	82	157.125	161.725	PUBLIC CORR. & PORT OPERATIONS
23		157.150	161.750	PUBLIC CORRESPONDENCE *ONLY* (TWO-FREQUENCY)
	83	157.175	161.775	
24		157.200	161.800	
	84	157.225	161.825	PUBLIC CORR. & PORT OPERATIONS
25		157.250	161.850	PUBLIC CORRESPONDENCE *ONLY* (TWO-FREQUENCY)
	85	157.275	161.875	
26		157.300	161.900	
	86	157.325	161.925	
27		157.350	161.950	
	87	157.375	161.975	
28		157.400	162.000	
	88	157.425	162.025	

4   Who can you talk to?

Other ships

Most vessels at sea are fitted with VHF – even some sailboards! You may talk to other vessels *on matters of ship's business* quite freely at any time. Marine VHF must not be used for idle chit-chat; if that is what you wish to do, use CB (Q11).

The usual procedure is to call the other vessel by name on Ch. 16, then switch to one of the designated *intership* channels by mutual agreement. The full procedure is given in chapter 7. Preferably, one of the *exclusive intership* channels should be used: Ch. 6, 8, 72 or 77. Note these particularly, as it is only with intership operation that *you* may have to make the choice!

It is quite permissible to contact another vessel directly on one of the intership working channels, by prior arrangement, without first calling on Ch. 16 (Q5). (Anything which reduces congestion on Ch. 16 has to be encouraged!)

Establishing contact with an unidentified vessel in sight can present a problem. The best way is to first establish communication by flashing light using the procedure on page 9 of the *International Code of Signals*, 1969, published by HMSO. Once communication has been established (you know the other vessel's call-sign and he knows yours), your message is, simply, 'K9'. This means 'I wish to communicate with you by VHF radiotelephony on Ch. 16'.

NOTE: Intership communication is *not permitted* while the ship is within, or within one mile of, any port, harbour, dock or anchorage in the territorial waters of any country – except in the case of distress, emergency involving danger to life or to navigation, for the purposes of safe navigation, or in the Port Operations Service. Intership communication *is* permitted on inland waterways provided that both vessels are under way.

Coastguards

Coastguards are concerned for your *safety* and you may talk to them on any aspect of safety quite freely at any time. All the major stations listen on Ch. 16, 24 hours a day, 365 days a year. Their names are the names of their location *plus* the word 'Coastguard', thus: 'Solent Coastguard', 'Dover Coastguard', etc.

After establishing contact on Ch. 16, British Coastguards will tell you to switch to Ch. 67 (Q5). The procedure for calling the Coastguard is given in chapter 8.

Below: A radio call to the lock control could save time when entering a yacht basin.

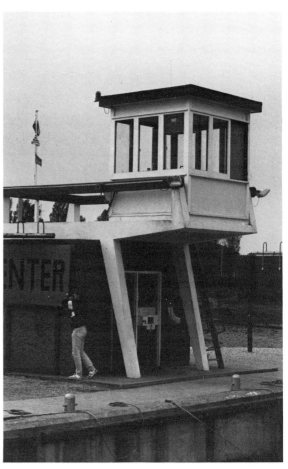

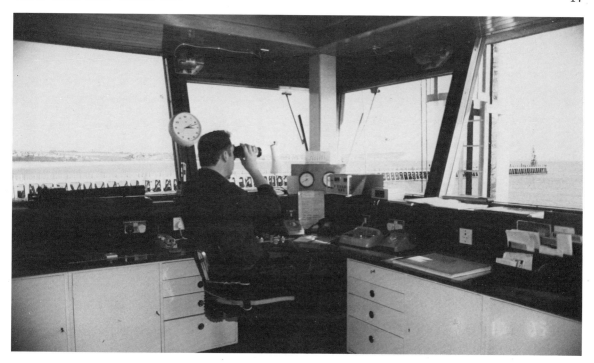

Above: Harbourmasters can provide valuable information, but contact procedure must be checked.

All the major British Coastguard Stations are now fitted with direction-finding equipment which operates on the VHF R/T channels. In case of difficulty, they may be able to give an indicated bearing upon request.

Harbourmasters

Most harbours throughout the world use VHF for providing harbour information. Many of them may be called, initially, on Ch. 16 and you will then be asked to switch to an appropriate Port Operations channel. The most popular are Channels 12 and 14, followed by 11 and 13, but many others are used. However, there are no general rules regarding the calling channel, the hours of watch or even the name to call! Some harbours listen only on their working channel, some listen only on Ch. 16. Others listen on both but prefer to be called directly on their working channel. Only the major ports maintain 24-hour watch; smaller harbours decide for themselves when they switch their sets on and off. There is no charge for communicating with a port or harbour.

Most harbours are addressed by their names *plus* the words 'Harbour Radio', thus: 'Cowes Harbour Radio', 'Langstone Harbour Radio', etc.

Many of the major ports, however, are addressed differently. Examples are: 'Mersey Radio' (for Liverpool), 'Long Room Port Control' (for Plymouth), 'VTS' (for Southampton) and 'Scarborough Lighthouse'. All British naval bases, which use Ch. 13, are addressed as 'Queen's Harbour Master' or 'QHM'. For full information, consult the *Admiralty List of Radio Signals,* Vol. 6. Available from all Admiralty chart agents, Part 1 covers Europe, Africa and most of Asia; Part 2 covers the rest of the world. Abridged information is published in the yachting almanacs.

Marinas and yacht clubs

For many years, British marinas and yacht clubs have shared the private frequency of 157.85 MHz called Channel 'M'. This is a private channel which may *only* be used for yacht club or marina business in Britain, Channel Islands and Isle of Man. Only *British yachts* may use this channel; the necessary authority is usually included with the yacht's Ship's Licence at no extra charge. On sets which cannot display the letter 'M', the number '37' or 'P1' may have to be selected. Some sets have a special button for Ch. M; consult the owner's

As Ch. M is not available to foreign yachts, the

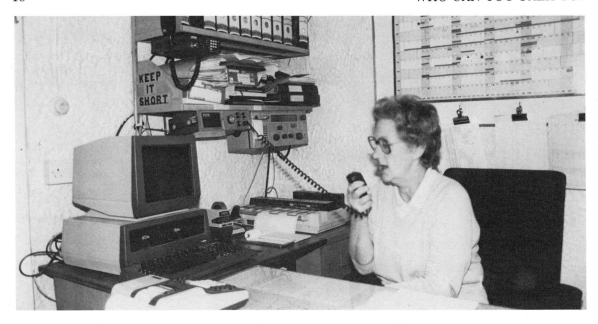

Above: British marinas and yacht clubs are only licensed to use Channels 80, 'M2' or 'M'.

DTI released Ch. 80 for use by British *marinas* in 1989 and it is hoped that this will soon become the primary channel. Also in 1989, the DTI released a second private channel, called 'M2', for use by British *yacht clubs*. The frequency is 161.425 MHz and this should become the principal channel when new sets are fitted. In some older sets, it can be programmed as 'P2'.

With one exception, British marinas and yacht clubs are *not authorised* for Ch. 16 and *must,* therefore, be *called directly* on Channels 80, M2 or M as appropriate.

The exception is Brighton Marina which may be addressed as 'Brighton Control' on Ch. 16 if Ch. M is not available on the yacht. On Ch. M, it is addressed as 'Brighton Marina'. On the Thames, St Katharine Yacht Haven must be called on Ch. 14 as 'St Katharines' and Brentford Dock Marina thus addressed also on Ch. 14.

Most French and Spanish marinas and yacht harbours use Ch. 09 *only*.

Apart from the exceptions given above, details of British yacht clubs and marinas are not given in the *Admiralty List of Radio Signals*. Details *are* given in the yachting almanacs but only when this is provided by the club or marina. British marinas are usually addressed by their name; yacht clubs by name *plus* the word 'Base', thus: 'Parkstone Base', 'Bosham Base', etc. There is no charge for communicating with a yacht club or marina.

Coast Radio Stations

These are usually operated by the telephone company/authority of the country concerned and form shore-side 'telephone exchanges' which connect ships with the worldwide telephone system. They also accept dictated telegrams. All Coast Radio Stations throughout the world can communicate in English. They are addressed by the name of their location *plus* the word 'Radio', thus: 'Niton Radio', 'Hastings Radio', etc.

Although most Coast Radio Stations listen continuously on Ch. 16 (the French *do not*), modern practice is to call directly on one of the station's working channels. Details of these and much more can be found in the *Admiralty List of Radio Signals* Vol. 1, of which Part 1 covers Europe, Africa and most of Asia, and Part 2 covers the rest of the world. Abridged information is also published in the yachting almanacs (Q14). An indication that a particular channel is engaged is given by hearing speech or a succession of 'pips' rather like the Greenwich 'pips' but slower. If neither speech nor 'pips' are heard, the channel is available for use (Q13,14). If a Coast Radio Station does not answer immediately, the 'pips' will be heard as soon as the microphone switch is released – provided that your transmission lasts at least six seconds. This indicates that your call has been received and a reply will be made soon.

The full procedure for obtaining a ship-to-shore telephone call is given in chapter 10.

Payment Although there is no charge for calling a Coast Radio Station, a charge is made for successful connection to the land-line. Throughout the UK there is only one standard charge – there are no peak rates or cheap rates.

Once communication with a Coast Radio Station has been established, the method of payment must be stated before the connection is made. This is done by stating your Accounting Authority Indicator Code (AAIC) or 'Account Code' for short.

There are several methods of payment. The cheapest is the 'YTD' system. This stands for Yacht Telephone Debit, and is a concession by British Telecom to allow the cost of a radiotelephone call to be directly debited to a home or office telephone account. To use this method, tell the Coast Radio Station 'My account code is YTD' *plus* the number to which you wish the call to be charged. This must include the area code. For example: 'My account code is YTD 01-234-5678'. The net cost of the call will then appear on the next quarterly bill for this number. In this way a crew-member or guest can make a telephone call and have it charged to his or her home telephone number.

The YTD system can *only* be used for calls from *British* yachts to *British* telephones via *British* Coast Radio Stations on VHF. If the call does not fulfil these requirements, an International Account Code Number must be given.

When application is made for a Ship's Radio Licence, an authorised accounting company must be appointed (from a selection offered) to handle the vessel's radio accounts. Merchant ships usually appoint the marine radio company which provides their radio equipment and, often, the Radio Officer(s). British yachts are advised to appoint British Telecom International PLC, whose AAIC is 'GB14'. When this code is given to a Coast Radio Station *anywhere in the world,* British Telecom send an entirely separate bill to the name and address which was given in paragraph 3 of the Ship's Licence application. A small handling charge will be added to the bill so, although 'GB14' *can* be used for British calls, the 'YTD' method is cheaper.

'Transferred Charge' (reversed charge) or 'collect' calls can be made provided the recipient agrees to accept the charge, which is the cost of the call plus two minutes.

In theory, calls via British Coast Radio Stations only can be charged to a credit card but this method is not advised. The card number may be overheard by an unscrupulous person who could use it for their own calls!

Relays A Coast Radio Station may be used as a 'relay station' between two vessels beyond 'line-of-sight' range. The charge equates, roughly, with that of a short-distance radio-telephone call. For example, a small yacht off Littlehampton could contact a friend anchored in Studland Bay via Niton Radio. The yacht off Littlehampton could also contact a friend sailing in the Clyde via Niton Radio, land-line and Clyde Radio – for which the charge would be higher. Taking this further, two vessels anywhere in the world can communicate with each other via the appropriate Coast Radio Stations and a land-line between. The charge depends on the distance involved between the two Coast Radio Stations.

Coast Radio Station broadcasts

In addition to *communicating* with individual vessels, Coast Radio Stations and many Coastguard stations *broadcast* vital information to shipping in general.

Gale warnings The appropriate Coast Radio Station broadcasts gale/storm warnings immediately upon receipt from the Meteorological Office (at Bracknell in the case of Britain). The initial announcement is given on Ch. 16 in the form:

SÉCURITÉ, SÉCURITÉ, SÉCURITÉ
ALL SHIPS, ALL SHIPS, ALL SHIPS
THIS IS (somewhere) RADIO,
   (somewhere) RADIO
FOR GALE WARNING, LISTEN
   (frequency and channel number)

The stated channel number should then be selected, and the gale warning is read out on that channel after a short interval. It is repeated on a six-hourly schedule until it is cancelled when the cancellation is also broadcast. For full information consult the *Admiralty List of Radio Signals,* Vol. 3.

As the major Coast Radio Stations broadcast simultaneously on the Medium Wave Band (around 2 MHz) as well as VHF, the initial announcement includes the Medium Wave frequency. This cannot be received on a marine VHF R/T set, so it should be ignored.

NOTE: The French word SÉCURITÉ (pronounced SAY-CURE-E-TAY), meaning 'safety', precedes all broadcasts of navigational importance to alert ships to this fact.

Navigational warnings Warnings of navigational hazards of a temporary nature such as wrecks, lights extinguished or radiobeacons inoperative are broadcast by the appropriate British Coast Radio Station every four hours on its broadcast working channel following an initial announcement on Ch. 16. All navigational warnings are preceded by the word 'SÉCURITÉ'.

British Coastguard Stations also broadcast Navigational Warnings on Ch. 67 following an announcement on Ch. 16. In the Dover Strait, Dover Coastguard broadcasts navigational information on Ch. 11 every H+40 (and H+55 in poor visibility). The French coastguard service for the English Channel (C.R.O.S.S.) broadcasts navigational information in English and French from Cap Gris Nez, Jobourg (Cherbourg Peninsula) and Ushant on Ch. 11 every half-hour (quarter-hour in poor visibility). For full information consult the *Admiralty List of Radio Signals*, Vol. 6, Part 1.

Weather forecasts British Coast Radio Stations broadcast the General Synopsis and Forecast for their own Sea Area and those immediately adjacent twice daily at fixed times in the morning and evening (varies with station). The forecast goes out on the main broadcast channel following an announcement on Ch. 16. Immediately after the first read-through, the information is repeated at dictation speed. Thus, not only is the information given at a more civilised hour than the Shipping Forecast on Radio 4, it is also much easier to copy by hand.

Jersey Radio broadcasts the General Synopsis and Forecast for the Channel Islands on request and five times a day at 0645, 0745, 1245, 1845 and 2245 on Ch. 25 and 82. Continental Coast Radio Stations also frequently broadcast gale warnings and weather forecasts. For full information, consult the *Admiralty List of Radio Signals*, Vol. 3 which covers the world. Note that although most Coast Radio Stations throughout the world broadcast gale warnings and weather messages in English, the French do not. All Met. broadcasts from French Coast Radio Stations and those of their territories and Tunisia are in the French language only.

In United States waters, the US Coastguard Stations frequently broadcast storm warnings and weather forecasts on the special Channel 22 CG. In this case, Ch. 22 is used as a *Single-frequency channel* with the shore station transmitting on the ship frequency of 157.1 MHz. European sets usually need modification to receive this frequency, or it may be programmed as a private channel if the set has the capacity. In highly-populated US coastal areas, taped weather messages are broadcast every four to six minutes on one of three private channel frequencies: 162.55 MHz (called 'WX1'), 162.4 MHz ('WX2') and 162.475 MHz ('WX3'); the messages are updated every two to three hours. These frequencies may also be programmed into some European sets; with the very latest sets they can be built in by the manufacturer.

In Canada, a similar continuous broadcast of weather information is made by the Coast Radio Stations on Chs. 21 or 83 according to location. Full information on these and USCG stations can be found in *ALRS*, Vol. 3.

Traffic lists Coast Radio Stations will accept telephone calls *from* the shore *to* a ship. The charge is the same either way. The procedure is to dial Freephone, 0800-378389 giving the boat's name, call-sign, voyage details and other information. These details are then passed to the appropriate Coast Radio Station which then calls the boat on Ch. 16. If answered immediately, the CRS dials the caller and makes the connection.

In the case of no reply, the boat's name and call-sign are then added to the Coast Radio Station's Traffic List. British stations broadcast their Traffic List 10 times between 0133 and 2233 (varies with station) together with other broadcasts such as Weather Forecasts, etc. The schedule of Traffic Lists is given in *ALRS*, Vol. 1.

Should you hear your vessel's name on a Traffic List, call the Coast Radio Station *on one of its working channels* and say 'What have you for me?' (Q13). The radio officer will then dial the caller's number and make the connection. The original caller still pays. The boat's name and call-sign are retained on the Traffic List for 24 hours; after that it is lost.

Right: A Coast Radio Station has aerials mounted on tall masts for maximum range.

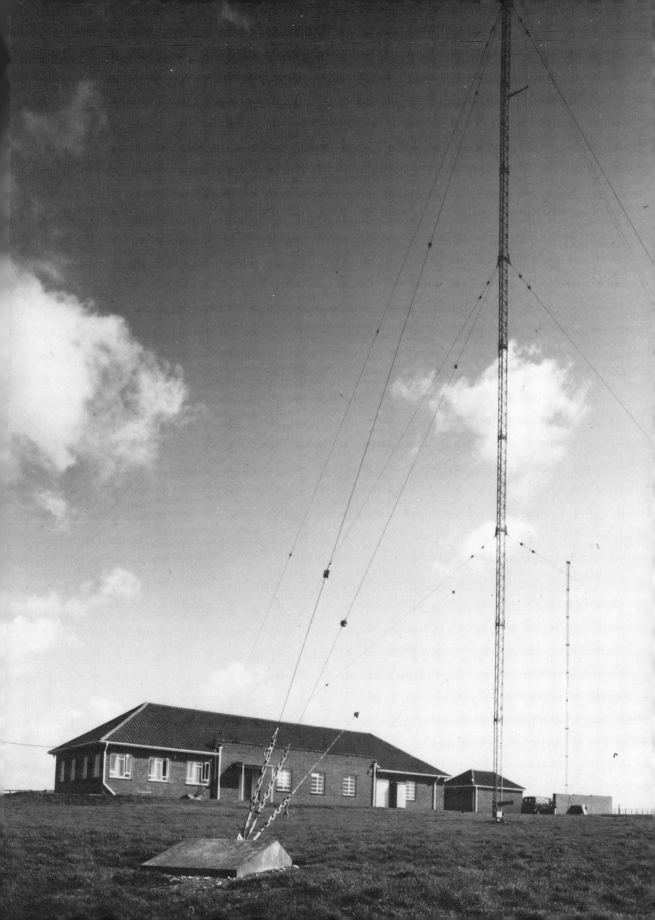

5 Some basic technicalities

Although no technical knowledge is required for the 'VHF Only' exam, as with the Driving Test, it is of great benefit to have a rough idea of some of the basic principles.

Simplex

The vast majority of radio communication stations operate in what is known as the Simplex mode. Inside, the box of electronics is divided into two parts. One is the *transmitter*, to which the microphone is connected for talking. The other is the *receiver*, to which is connected the loudspeaker or earpiece for listening. Both share the same power supply (usually a 12 V battery) and both require an aerial or antenna. The same aerial can be used for transmission or reception – but *not both at the same time*. So with a Simplex installation, you have to decide whether to use your set for talking *or* listening since you cannot do both at once.

The change-over is achieved with a spring-loaded *press-to-talk* (PTT) switch fitted to the hand microphone or concealed in the handle of a telephone-type handset. With the set switched on and the PTT switch in the released position, the set is in the listening mode. To make a transmission, the PTT switch must be pressed and held pressed all the time you are talking. The PTT switch must then be released to listen. This may sound inconvenient but, with a few minutes' practice, the 'press-to-talk, release-to-listen' habit is quickly acquired.

As the name implies, the Simplex system keeps the equipment simple and inexpensive, although it is not quite as easy as operating a normal domestic telephone. It also requires the co-operation of the other person, since they must wait for you to finish speaking before they can reply. Having said something, therefore, you say 'OVER' just before releasing the PTT switch to indicate to the other person that you are about to pass the channel 'over' to them.

This works well between two people who are versed in this one-way-at-a-time system, but it can be a little daunting for a completely uninitiated person such as a ship's passenger telephoning a person ashore.

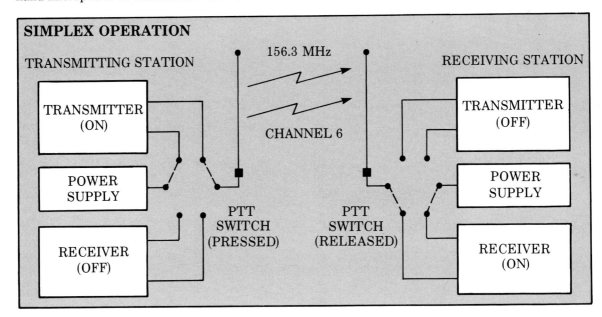

SIMPLEX OPERATION

TRANSMITTING STATION   156.3 MHz   RECEIVING STATION

TRANSMITTER (ON)

POWER SUPPLY

RECEIVER (OFF)

CHANNEL 6

PTT SWITCH (PRESSED)

PTT SWITCH (RELEASED)

TRANSMITTER (OFF)

POWER SUPPLY

RECEIVER (ON)

Duplex

This system allows for simultaneous transmission and reception so that an ordinary two-way conversation may be carried out between a vessel and a telephone ashore.

Unless an electronic switching device is used, two separate aerials are needed: one for the transmitter and a second for the receiver. To operate on the same frequency these must be widely separated – if they were not, most of the transmitted power would be picked up by the receiving aerial and probably damage the receiver. On a small ship, however, the two aerials can never be very far apart.

The problem is reduced by arranging for the two stations to transmit on two completely different, widely-separated frequencies. The ship's receiver is tuned to the signal from the shore transmitter and, similarly, the shore receiver is tuned to pick up the signal from the ship. Even with two different frequencies, a good separation must still be maintained between the transmitting and receiving aerials, otherwise the transmission may overcome the frequency separation.

All Coast Radio Stations are equipped for Duplex operation; this is why all the public correspondence channels are two-frequency channels. It should now be clear why the two-frequency channels cannot possibly be used for intership communication. On Ch. 04, for example, *all* ships transmit on 156.2 MHz and listen on 160.8 MHz. Not only can you not hear yourself (there is no need), no other ship can hear you either! (Q14).

'Semi-duplex'

The average yacht's Simplex R/T set may be used for telephone calls to the shore via Coast Radio Stations provided the set has some, if not all, of the two-frequency channels, and assuming the caller on the yacht has the co-operation of the person ashore. Although the latter can speak and listen simultaneously, the person afloat cannot: the person ashore should be advised of this beforehand, for this will save a good deal of confusion, explanation, time and money if you need to make a call.

Range

VHF radio waves travel in straight lines, just like rays of light radiating from a lighthouse. In the same way, the range is restricted by the curvature of the earth. Provided sufficient power is transmitted (and 25 watts (Q7) is about ten times the minimum required), the aerial-to-aerial range is determined by the height of the respective aerials above sea level (asl).

As the VHF wave behaves like an invisible beam of light, the tables used for determining the extreme range of a light at sea can also be used for determining the range of a VHF signal. In *Reed's*

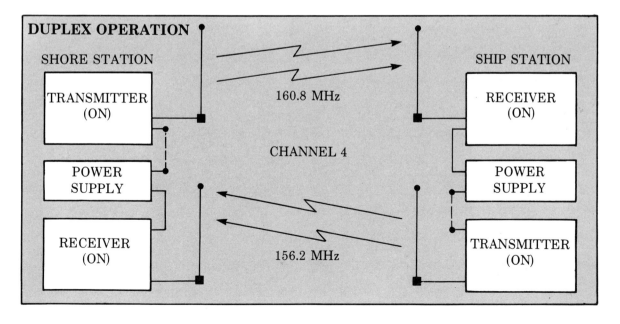

DUPLEX OPERATION

SHORE STATION

TRANSMITTER (ON)

POWER SUPPLY

RECEIVER (ON)

160.8 MHz

CHANNEL 4

156.2 MHz

SHIP STATION

RECEIVER (ON)

POWER SUPPLY

TRANSMITTER (ON)

the extreme range is referred to as the 'Distance Off Lights Just Seen or Dipping'. To use the table in this way, simply enter the height of one aerial as the 'Height of Light' and that of the other aerial as the 'Height of Eye' (it does not matter in which order the aerials are taken). The junction of the two columns gives the range in nautical miles. As the VHF wave is refracted (bent) towards the Earth slightly more than light, the figure thus obtained may be increased by ten per cent for maximum accuracy. However, accepting the figure as quoted – often referred to as 'line-of-sight' range – gives a little to spare for safety.

In the absence of tables, the range under any circumstances is easily calculated if you have a pocket calculator. For *each* aerial, the range in nautical miles to the 'radio horizon' (slightly greater than the visible horizon) is given by the formula $R = 2.25\sqrt{h}$, where h is the height of the *centre* of the aerial above sea level in metres. The two ranges thus obtained are then added to give the total aerial-to-aerial range. For example, two cabin cruisers or small fishing boats, both with aerials at 3m (10ft) asl would have a horizon range as follows:

$R = 2.25 \sqrt{h}$
$R = 2.25 \sqrt{3}$
$R = 2.25 \times 1.73$
$R = 3.9$ nautical miles for *each* aerial

Thus, their boat-to-boat range would be $3.9 + 3.9 = 7.8$ nautical miles *only*. No increase in power would increase the range; remember that the VHF signal is like a light at sea – no matter how powerful the light, it is invisible below the horizon!

The 'rag-and-stick' sailor with an aerial at the top of his mast fares much better. Even a small yacht's aerial would be 10m asl, giving a horizon-range of just over seven nautical miles or 14¼ miles boat-to-boat. This is nearly twice that between two power boats. *These are typical boat-to-boat ranges.*

Much greater distances can be achieved by all vessels to shore stations which can put their aerials on tall masts on high ground. For example, a small yacht with an aerial at 10m asl can communicate with a shore station with an aerial at 100m asl at the following range:

$R = 2.25 \sqrt{h} + 2.25 \sqrt{h}$
$R = 2.25 \sqrt{10} + 2.25 \sqrt{100}$
$R = 2.25 \times 3.16 + 2.25 \times 10$
$R = 7.12 + 22.5$
$R = 29.62$
say 30 nautical miles (Q4)

Capture effect

Marine VHF uses the system of Frequency Modulation (FM). The end result is much the same as that produced by Amplitude Modulation (AM), as used on the Medium Wave and Short Wave Bands, but an important feature of FM is that the receiver can only reproduce one signal at any one time. If several signals are being received at once, the FM receiver 'locks-on' to the strongest signal and reproduces it to the complete exclusion of all others (Q4). As a result, you never hear the unintelligible jumble of voices typical of the Medium Wave Band at night when Continental stations are strong. This, plus the fact that the 25 watts allowed is grossly in excess of the minimum required to achieve the fairly short range, ensures that marine VHF signals tend to be mostly 'loud and clear' or nothing!

It is for this reason that a low-power (1W) switch is fitted to the transmitter section of all marine VHF sets with an output power in excess of 1W. To avoid causing unnecessary interference to other stations, the minimum amount of power should always be used (Q7). This benefits the users also, as it saves battery power. (The average Marine VHF draws about ⅓ amp on receive, 1 amp on low-power transmit and 5-6 amps on high-power transmit).

Low power should always be used for the short-range inter-ship communication and for communicating with local harbour masters, yacht clubs and marinas. Full power will not be of any benefit, and will only cause interference to other stations some distance away (Q7).

Low power will also suffice for routine calls when in sight of a Coastguard Station but any Distress or Urgency calls should, of course, be made on full power. Full power should also be used for telephone calls via Coast Radio Stations, who like to put a strong signal down the line.

Dual watch

Most modern marine VHF sets of the 'fully-synthesised' 55-channel type feature an extremely useful facility known as dual watch. This is a circuit which *effectively* (though not actually) enables the set to receive on two channels at the same time: Channel 16 (which has priority) and any one of the remaining 54 channels as selected.

In dual-watch mode, the receiver switches continuously (scans) between the channel

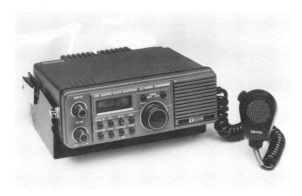

Above: A typical VHF set for installation in a boat. Note the PTT switch on the microphone.

selected and Ch. 16, spending most time on the selected channel. Should a transmission be received on the working channel, it will be heard with fair clarity although, since the receiver will continue to scan Ch.16 momentarily, the odd syllable may be missed. If this happens, the dual watch facility may be switched off to allow uninterrupted reception on the working channel.

If a signal is received on Ch. 16 with dual watch in operation, the receiver will 'lock-on' to it *and remain on Ch. 16 during the whole transmission.* Thus 100 per cent of transmissions on Ch. 16 and 90 per cent of transmissions on the selected channel will be received.

This feature is especially useful if private calling arrangements have been made. Although it is usual to make the initial contact with other vessels on Ch. 16, it is quite acceptable to call directly on an inter-ship working channel (06, 08, 72 or 77) at a pre-arranged time by private agreement (Q5). By using dual watch, a listening watch may then be kept on Ch. 16 as well as the pre-arranged channel (Q4).

Always switch off dual watch before transmitting. Some sets transmit on Ch. 16 when in dual watch mode, some on the working channel; the most up-to-date sets will not transmit at all.

Squelch

Because of the enormous amount of signal amplification which occurs in a VHF receiver, a great deal of noise (hash) is generated which can be very objectionable between signals. When a signal is received, it over-rides the noise so only the signal is heard but, between signals, you get a loud hiss. The squelch circuit combats this by muting the loudspeaker in the absence of a signal so the hiss is not heard. As soon as a signal is received, however, the muting system is overridden, enabling the signal to be heard (Q7).

For best results the squelch control should be turned off (fully anti-clockwise) then advanced slowly until the hiss *just* stops. If it is advanced too far, the sensitivity of the receiver will be reduced so much that weak signals may be missed. The setting will not vary as the channels or volume control are adjusted, but it may vary slightly with fluctuations in battery voltage and it may get knocked, so check the setting frequently.

Selcall

The Selcall (Selective Calling) system enables a Coast Radio Station to call an individual ship, not by calling out the name on Ch. 16 but by playing a short electronically-generated tune (Q4). Every ship which participates in this scheme is allocated a 'signature tune' which is decoded in the receiver. The receiver then flashes lights and/or sounds a warning, and also records the fact that the set has been called. Some decoders also record the indentification of the calling station. Although little used for yachts, the system could be useful if you wish to leave your yacht for a short period. Upon your return, the set would indicate whether or not it had been called in the meantime without you having to wait nearly two hours for the next Traffic List.

Test call

An extremely useful and inexpensive optional extra, easily fitted to all sets, is an output test meter which gives a direct indication of the transmitted output power without having to rely on a friend or Coastguard for a 'radio check'. The more sophisticated devices also indicate the efficiency of the aerial and cable, enabling the performance of the whole transmitter/aerial system to be measured every time the transmit switch is pressed. Very reassuring.

It takes ten seconds to complete the test and this is the maximum time allowed if you are not in communication with someone (Q4). If you are making a test transmission without addressing another station, you must still announce your identification in the usual way, even though you are not addressing anyone.

6 Priority of signals on Channel 16

In general, initial contact with other stations is made on Channel 16. However, as Ch. 16 is also used for distress and other emergency calls, a scale of priorities has been established.

Distress signals

Top priority for the use of Ch. 16 is given to distress signals. A distress situation is indicated by the use of the word 'MAYDAY'. This indicates that the *vessel* (or aircraft) is in *grave* and *imminent* danger, that is to say *sinking* (or about to sink) or *on fire* (Q1). Under these circumstances it might be thought that 'Mayday' is a silly word to say – but it is not what it seems. Although English is the international language of radio, all the procedural words, or *prowords* as they are termed, are French. So, if you get into difficulties, you cry for help in French! The French spell it *'m'aidez'* meaning literally 'come to my aid' or in basic English, 'HELP'!

The distress signal is very special for two reasons. It is a *broadcast* – it is not addressed to anyone in particular – and it is the only occasion on which *messages are exchanged* on Ch. 16. Consequently, whenever there is a distress situation, *radio silence is automatically imposed throughout the whole operation*. An announcement that normal or restricted working may be resumed on Ch. 16 will be made, on Ch. 16, by the station controlling distress communications. This may be the distressed vessel itself but is more likely to be a Coastguard Station or possibly a Coast Radio Station. For this reason *it is vital to keep listening on Channel 16* to keep abreast of the current situation. The procedure for a Mayday broadcast, which must be *authorised* (but not necessarily made) by the *master* of the vessel, is given in chapter 11.

Urgent calls

All emergency calls apart from sinking or fire are prefixed by the prowords 'PAN-PAN' (Q12). This again is derived from the French *en panne*

meaning 'in difficulty' and takes second priority to distress. *It is not a cry for help.* It is simply a plea for radio priority: radio silence is observed during the message and for three minutes after. As it is not a broadcast, the 'PAN-PAN' message must be addressed to someone. Usually it will be addressed to a Coastguard Station but, if the vessel is out of range of the shore, the message may be addressed to 'All Ships'.

A variation, 'PAN-PAN MEDICO', is used to prefix calls to British Coast Radio Stations requesting urgent (and free) medical advice (Q12). The procedure for obtaining medical advice via foreign Coast Radio Stations is given in the *Admiralty List of Radio Signals,* Vol. 1.

Short 'PAN-PAN' messages may be broadcast to 'All Ships' on Ch. 16, but a Coastguard Station will ask a vessel to switch to a working channel: Ch. 67 in Britain (Q5).

Safety Calls

Broadcast warnings of strong winds and navigational hazards by Coast Radio Stations and Coastguard Stations are prefixed by the proword 'SÉCURITÉ' (pronounced 'say-cure-ee-tay') which is French for 'safety'. As yachts do not broadcast, no procedure is given in these pages. However, if you wish to advise a Coastguard Station of a newly-found navigational hazard, the initial call could be preceded by the word 'SÉCURITÉ'.

Other priorities

In all, there are ten internationally-agreed priorities listed in the *BTI Handbook for Radio Operators* but the above are the most important.

Routine calls

Provided none of the above situations are in operation, routine calls may be made on Ch. 16. The procedure for calling different stations is given in the following pages.

7 Routine call to another vessel

This is probably the most common use of the VHF/RT set. It is also the easiest procedure. As you will normally be calling someone you know or can see, it is usual to use vessel names rather than call-signs (Q10). However, call-signs can be used if known in case of difficulty or duplication of names (Q10). Many yachts now display the call-sign on the dodger for easy identification and this is strongly recommended. The author had the call-sign sewn onto the mainsail in two-foot high letters, and on the mizzen in 18-inch high letters;

they could be seen from more than a mile away with good binoculars!

Although the usual procedure is to make the initial call on Ch. 16, it is quite permissible to call directly on one of the intership channels (06, 08, 72 or 77) by prior arrangement (Q5).

As an example, with yacht *Gaffer* calling another *Flash,* it will be assumed that the initial call is being made on Ch. 16 as this is the usual case. Having made quite sure that Ch. 16 is quiet, *Gaffer* presses the press-to-talk button:

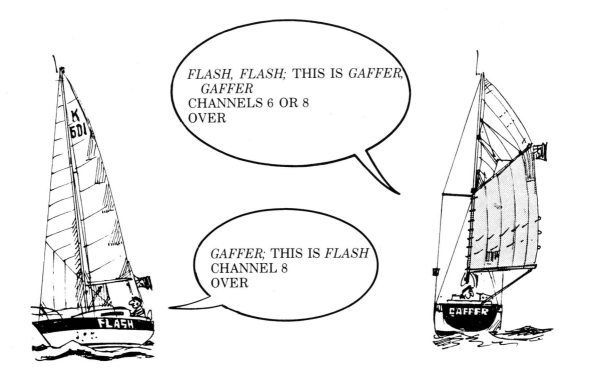

Before switching channels, it is *vital* that the calling station confirms the working channel:

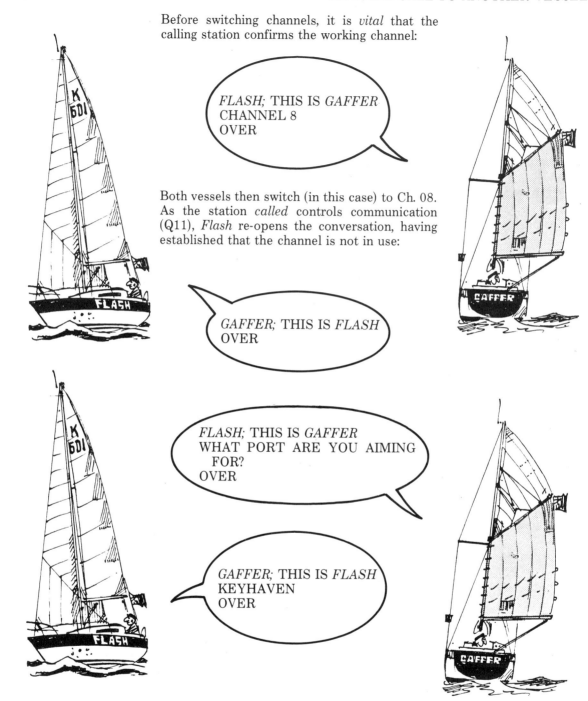

FLASH; THIS IS *GAFFER*
CHANNEL 8
OVER

Both vessels then switch (in this case) to Ch. 08. As the station *called* controls communication (Q11), *Flash* re-opens the conversation, having established that the channel is not in use:

GAFFER; THIS IS *FLASH*
OVER

FLASH; THIS IS *GAFFER*
WHAT PORT ARE YOU AIMING
    FOR?
OVER

GAFFER; THIS IS *FLASH*
KEYHAVEN
OVER

The exchange can continue as long as *necessary* (Q11) with each station saying '*Flash;* this is *Gaffer*' or '*Gaffer;* this is *Flash*' every time the microphone button is pressed (Q10). At the end of the exchange of messages, the usual 'goodbye'

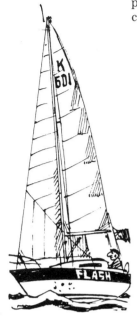

pleasantries can be exchanged but, finally, the communication is closed as follows:

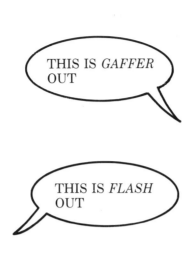

> THIS IS *GAFFER*
> OUT

> THIS IS *FLASH*
> OUT

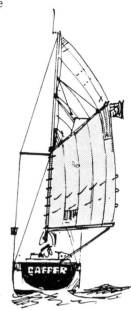

Both stations then switch back to Ch.16, ready for any further calls.

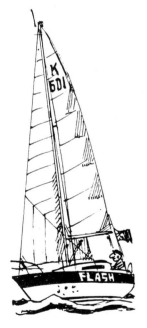

If the initial call is made directly on an intership working channel (06, 08, 72 or 77), the procedure can be shortened as follows:

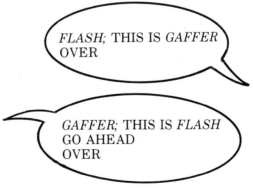

> *FLASH;* THIS IS *GAFFER*
> OVER

> *GAFFER;* THIS IS *FLASH*
> GO AHEAD
> OVER

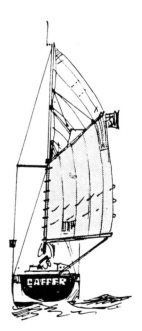

In the case of direct calling on an intership channel, the dual watch facility can prove invaluable as it enables a vessel to maintain listening watch on a working channel in addition to Channel 16 (Q4).

8 To call coastguards

The prime task of Her Majesty's Coastguards is safety of life at sea but they also have a secondary task to co-ordinate pollution control operations. Contrary to popular belief, they are not now concerned about contraband and have not been for the past 150 years!

The Coastguards are a civil, uniformed service of the Department of Transport and operate a chain of strategically-placed Coastguard Stations all round the UK coastline. Although most have a view of the sea, visibility in UK waters is rarely good so great reliance is placed on VHF Radiotelephony. So, although there are now many fewer Coastguards manning Lookouts (as they were called) than there were some years ago, the service is now very much better than it was. Only a few years ago, you were lucky if a Coastguard could *see* you three miles away; now he or she can *hear* you 30 miles away! For this reason it is now most important that everyone who goes to sea carries a VHF radiotelephone.

Coastguard Station weather broadcasts			
Aberdeen	0320	Portland	0220
Belfast	0305	Shetland	0105
Brixham	0050	Solent	0040
Clyde	0020	Stornoway	0110
Dover	0105	Swansea	0005
Falmouth	0140	Thames	0010
Forth	0205	Tyne-Tees	0150
Holyhead	0235	Yarmouth	0040
Humber	0340		
Liverpool	0210		
Milford Haven	0335		
Oban	0240		
Pentland	0135		

The above are starting times: the broadcast is repeated every four hours following the time given.

Weather forecasts

In addition to acting as communication centres, Coastguard Stations also regularly broadcast weather forecasts, strong wind warnings and local navigational warnings on Ch. 67 after a preliminary announcement on Ch. 16. The table on this page gives the starting time (local) for HMCG weather broadcasts. These are then repeated at four-hourly intervals, or two-hourly intervals if a gale warning or strong wind warning is in force.

Navigational help

For the Dover Strait, Dover Coastguard broadcasts a 'Channel Navigation Information Service' on Ch.11 at H+40 during fine weather and again at H+55 during poor visibility, following an initial announcement on Ch. 16. Their French counterparts, Gris Nez Traffic, Jobourg Traffic and Ouessant Traffic (Ushant) do the same in English and French on Ch. 11.

Dover Coastguard controls radar stations at St Margaret's Bay and Dungeness. Vessels within range of these stations can ask for a range and bearing from either by calling Dover Coastguard on Ch. 80.

Most UK Coastguard Stations can now give the *bearing* (but not *range*) of a station calling on VHF. By 'crossing' two such bearings, say from Portland Coastguard and Solent Coastguard, a fair 'fix' can be obtained. The bearings have an accuracy of plus or minus two degrees at best, so the system is not highly accurate. In poor visibility after a long and hard trip across the Channel, though, such a fix will be far better than an estimated position or one obtained by dead reckoning. Although primarily intended for use in an emergency situation, the service is freely available for anyone who *needs* it. Obviously the Coastguards cannot cope with 5,000 yachtsmen in the Solent area each calling for a bearing every half-hour on a sunny afternoon, so the service must not be abused.

Calling procedure for routine calls

The yacht *Gaffer* (call-sign MABC) approaching Torbay and wishing for a report of the sea conditions there, would call Brixham Coastguard on Ch. 16:

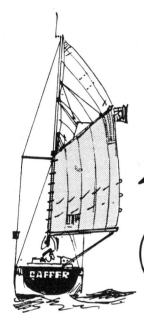

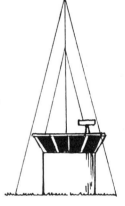

> BRIXHAM COASTGUARD,
> BRIXHAM COASTGUARD, THIS IS
> MIKE ALPHA BRAVO CHARLIE,
> MIKE ALPHA BRAVO CHARLIE
> SAFETY MESSAGE; CHANNEL
> SIX SEVEN
> OVER

> MIKE ALPHA BRAVO CHARLIE,
> THIS IS BRIXHAM COAST-
> GUARD
> CHANNEL SIX SEVEN AND STAND
> BY
> OVER

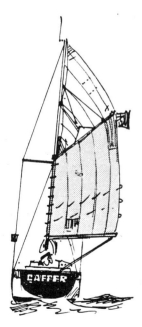

> BRIXHAM COASTGUARD, THIS IS
> MIKE ALPHA BRAVO CHARLIE
> CHANNEL SIX SEVEN AND STAN-
> DING BY
> OVER

Both stations then switch to Ch. 67 (Q5) and the yacht waits for the Coastguard to re-open communication:

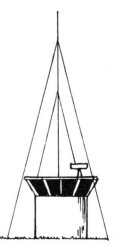

> MIKE ALPHA BRAVO CHARLIE,
> THIS IS BRIXHAM COAST-
> GUARD
> WHAT HAVE YOU FOR ME
> OVER

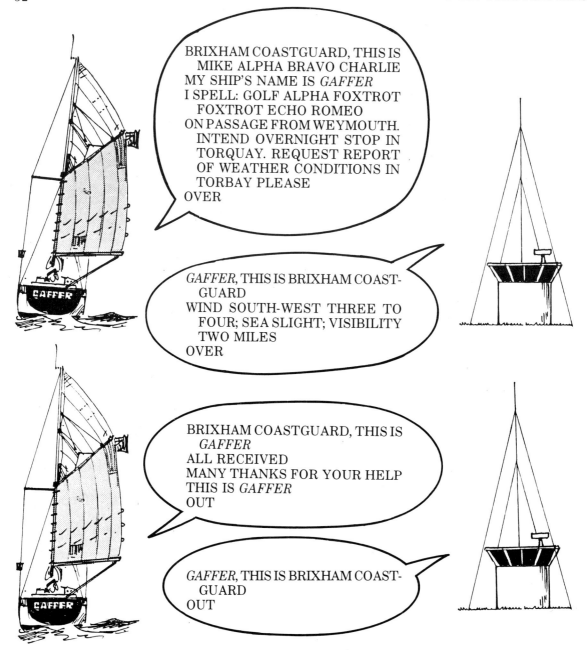

BRIXHAM COASTGUARD, THIS IS
MIKE ALPHA BRAVO CHARLIE
MY SHIP'S NAME IS *GAFFER*
I SPELL: GOLF ALPHA FOXTROT
FOXTROT ECHO ROMEO
ON PASSAGE FROM WEYMOUTH.
INTEND OVERNIGHT STOP IN
TORQUAY. REQUEST REPORT
OF WEATHER CONDITIONS IN
TORBAY PLEASE
OVER

GAFFER, THIS IS BRIXHAM COAST-
GUARD
WIND SOUTH-WEST THREE TO
FOUR; SEA SLIGHT; VISIBILITY
TWO MILES
OVER

BRIXHAM COASTGUARD, THIS IS
GAFFER
ALL RECEIVED
MANY THANKS FOR YOUR HELP
THIS IS *GAFFER*
OUT

GAFFER, THIS IS BRIXHAM COAST-
GUARD
OUT

Even a short conversation such as this looks very longwinded in print but, in practice, the whole episode would probably be over in two or three minutes.

You will notice that *every* transmission starts with the name of the station being *called*, followed immediately by the call-sign or name of the *calling* station – twice for the initial call (Q10). In the case of ship-to-shore communication, the *shore station* controls communication, that is dictates the working channel (Q11). In the case of ship-to-ship communication, it is the *station called* which controls communication (Q11).

If no reply is received to an initial call, the calling station *must* wait three minutes before making another attempt (Q11). Remember that, except in the case of distress, calls on Ch. 16 must not last longer than one minute (Q6).

Weather forecasts

In addition to the regular four-hourly (or two-hourly) weather broadcasts, British Coastguards will repeat the forecast at any time upon request. However, they do become irate with people who call for a repetition of the forecast just after or before a broadcast. Since these broadcasts are interspersed with those of the Coast Radio Stations, BBC Radio 4 on 200kHz and local BBC/IBA radio stations, there is very little excuse for calling for a special, personal repetition.

Radio checks

As the transmitter section of the average marine VHF set has no in-built means of testing, most Coastguards (but *not* Solent Coastguard) will confirm that your transmitter is working correctly. The procedure on Ch. 16 is as follows:

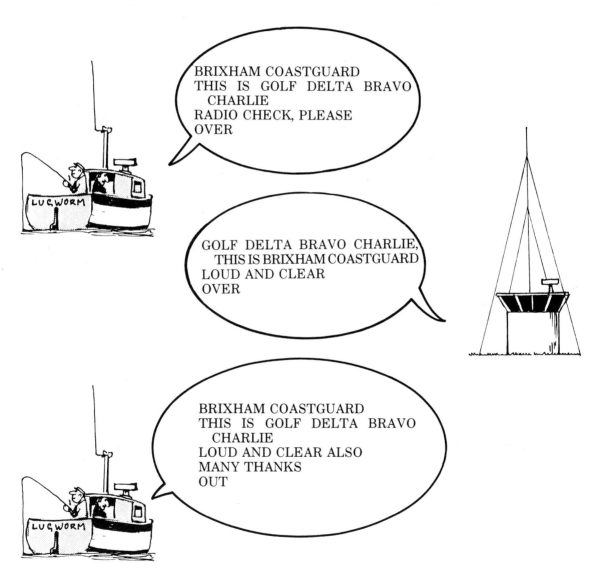

> BRIXHAM COASTGUARD
> THIS IS GOLF DELTA BRAVO
>   CHARLIE
> RADIO CHECK, PLEASE
> OVER

> GOLF DELTA BRAVO CHARLIE,
>   THIS IS BRIXHAM COASTGUARD
> LOUD AND CLEAR
> OVER

> BRIXHAM COASTGUARD
> THIS IS GOLF DELTA BRAVO
>   CHARLIE
> LOUD AND CLEAR ALSO
> MANY THANKS
> OUT

Coastguards often acknowledge this final transmission with a couple of quick presses of the microphone button without saying anything.

Local variations

Normally, the initial call to a Coastguard Station would be made on Ch. 16 (Q5) but procedure is easier and quicker with Dover Coastguard who will accept initial calls directly on Ch. 80 for navigational information. As this channel is used for communicating with merchant ships and is a two-frequency channel (from-ship calls cannot be heard), *wait three minutes* (Q11) if your first call is not answered.

Urgent calls

Any calls concerning difficulty such as dismasting, engine failure, lack of fuel, rudder problems, man overboard or diving accidents, should be addressed to a Coastguard by preceding what would otherwise have been a routine call on Ch. 16 by the phrase 'PAN-PAN, PAN-PAN, PAN-PAN'.

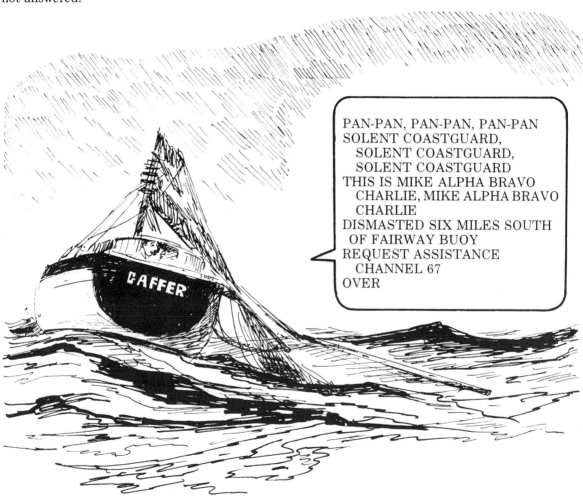

> PAN-PAN, PAN-PAN, PAN-PAN
> SOLENT COASTGUARD,
>   SOLENT COASTGUARD,
>   SOLENT COASTGUARD
> THIS IS MIKE ALPHA BRAVO
>   CHARLIE, MIKE ALPHA BRAVO
>   CHARLIE
> DISMASTED SIX MILES SOUTH
>   OF FAIRWAY BUOY
> REQUEST ASSISTANCE
>   CHANNEL 67
> OVER

No doubt Solent Coastguard would then ask *Gaffer* to change to Ch. 67 to ask for further details.

This type of mishap raises a question. How did *Gaffer* talk to Solent Coastguard with his aerial several feet under water at the top of his mast? The answer is that, being a prudent yachtsman, the owner would not dream of going to sea without a VHF set *and* an emergency aerial!

9 To call yacht clubs, marinas and Port Radio Stations

For many years, British yacht clubs have shared the private channel 'M' on 157.85 MHz with British marinas. From 1990, however, it is hoped that an increasing number of British yacht clubs will change to the new, exclusive private channel 'M2' on 161.425 MHz. No British yacht clubs are allowed on Ch. 16 so they *must* be called directly on Ch. M2 or Ch. M. Try M2 first (if fitted in your set), then Ch. M if there is no reply. Address the club by name (usually 'Somewhere Base') then identify yourself by *boat's name* just like calling another boat on a working channel (p29). For example: 'Bosham Base, Bosham Base; this is Flash, Flash. OVER'.

Marinas

In the past, British marinas have shared Ch. M with British yacht clubs but many are now changing to the recently-released International Channel 80 to enable them to communicate with foreign yachts as well as British yachts. With one exception (Brighton), marinas are not allowed on Ch. 16 and *must* be called directly on Ch. 80 or Ch. M. Try Ch. 80 first; if there is no reply after three minutes, try again on Ch. M. Brighton Marina may be addressed as 'Brighton Control' on Ch. 16 if Ch. M is not available; yacht harbours in the Thames must be called on Ch. 14. Much information can be found in the popular yachting almanacs, of which the *Cruising Almanac* published by *Practical Boat Owner* is the most comprehensive. Most French and Spanish yacht harbours seem to operate on Ch. 09 *only*.

Port Radio Stations

Most decent, self-respecting harbourmasters throughout the world have a VHF/RT station and welcome calls from yachts. Although there is no compulsion for yachts to ask permission to enter or leave harbour in most cases (at Dover there is!), it is only common courtesy and costs nothing.

Before calling a Port or Harbour Radio Station, however, it is vital to check all the station's details in the *Admiralty List of Radio Signals*, Vol. 6, as all ports and harbours differ.

Local variations

Most harbours are addressed as '(somewhere) Harbour Radio' but most of the major ports are not. If the station is *not* addressed as '(somewhere) Harbour Radio', the form of address is in *ALRS* Vol. 6.

Although all Coast Radio Stations and Coastguard Stations work 24 hours per day, few harbours do. The hours of watch are detailed in *ALRS* Vol. 6.

Calling channels differ. Some harbours/ports listen only on Ch. 16; some listen only on their working channel and some listen on both! Again, see *ALRS* Vol. 6 for details. Whenever possible, the initial call should be made on the port's working channel. (Q6). (At some future date, initial calls to *all* shore stations will be made on their working channel).

By far the most common port operations working channels are Ch. 12 and Ch. 14 but there are many others. Check first (*ALRS* Vol. 6) to ensure that your set has the working channel(s) of the harbour/port concerned.

For example, if the yacht *Gaffer* in chapter 8 came within the shelter of Torbay between 0900-1300, 1400-1700 and 1800-2200 (local time) any day of the week or weekend from the beginning of May until the end of September – the hours of watch of the Port Radio Station at Torquay – she could switch to Ch. 14 and call them up:

TORQUAY HARBOUR RADIO
TORQUAY HARBOUR RADIO
THIS IS *GAFFER, GAFFER*
CALL-SIGN MIKE, ALPHA, BRAVO,
   CHARLIE
OVER

If the call is to a predominantly commercial harbour or major port, it helps to identify the vessel calling as 'yacht . . . ' in the initial radio message.

10   Ship-to-shore telephone calls

Coast Radio Stations act as shore-side 'telephone exchanges' to connect vessels with the world-wide telephone system or accept dictated radio-telegrams. They cannot give you harbour information (except for Jersey Radio and St Peter Port Radio, which can) and they are not particularly interested in your safety. They are the first shore stations to be converted to the 'direct calling' system so, although most still listen on Ch. 16 (the French do not!), *the initial call should be made directly on any of their working channels.*

Procedure

1.   Write down the telephone number you wish to call.
2.   Decide on the method of payment. If you wish to use the 'YTD' system and have the cost of the call directly debited to a British telephone number, write that down too. If the call is *not* to a British telephone, via a British Coast Radio Station on VHF, your Account Code is 'GB14' for British Telecom.
3.   Find out the Coast Radio Station's working channels, in *ALRS* Vol. 1 or yachting almanacs, then switch from channel to channel to find one which is available for use. This will be indicated by complete silence, that is no speech, dialling tone or 'pips'. (Q13, Q14).
4.   Having found a free channel, *switch to high power,* hold the microphone close to your mouth, press the microphone switch and *slowly* say:

> (somewhere) RADIO
> (somewhere) RADIO
> THIS IS (call-sign) (call-sign)
> ONE (YTD) TELEPHONE CALL, PLEASE
> OVER

Then release the microphone switch. If the Coast Radio Station does not acknowledge immediately, the 'pips' will be heard. This indicates *to you* that your call has been registered and indicates *to everyone else* that the channel is now engaged.

Wait on this channel until the Coast Radio Station answers. The Coast Radio Station will acknowledge by saying either:

> WHO IS CALLING (somewhere) RADIO ON CHANNEL X?

or alternatively:

> (your call-sign)
> THIS IS (somewhere) RADIO
> WHAT HAVE YOU FOR ME?
> OVER

5.   With the microphone close to your mouth, press the microphone switch and *slowly* say:

> (somewhere) RADIO
> THIS IS (call-sign)
> MY SHIP'S NAME IS (name)
> I SPELL (phonetics)
> I HAVE A CALL FOR (number to be called)
> MY ACCOUNT CODE IS (YTD plus Area Code and number of telephone account to be debited *or*, simply, GOLF BRAVO ONE FOUR)
> OVER

Then release the microphone switch. The Coast Radio Station will reply saying:

> (ship's name)
> THIS IS (somewhere) RADIO
> TRYING TO CONNECT YOU
> STAND BY, PLEASE
> OVER

6.   Press the microphone switch and say:

> (somewhere) RADIO
> THIS IS (ship's name)
> STANDING BY
> OVER

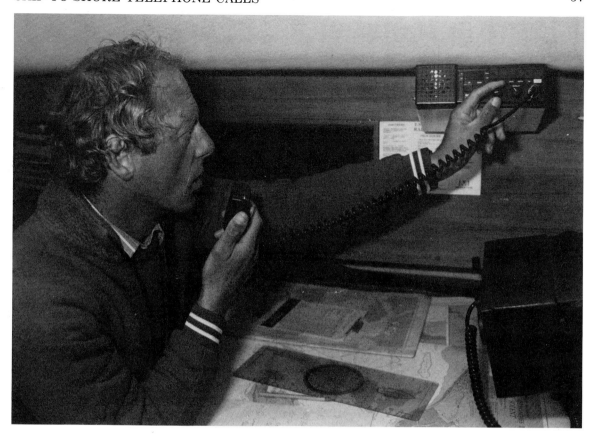

Above: When making a telephone call make sure you have all the details worked out beforehand.

Then release the microphone switch. When your correspondent answers the telephone, the Coast Radio Station will say:

> (ship's name)
> THIS IS (somewhere) RADIO
> GO AHEAD NOW, YOU ARE CONNECTED
> OVER

7.   Now you can press the microphone switch and speak to your correspondent. With a Simplex set, you must release the microphone switch *each time* you stop talking, as you cannot hear your correspondent as long as your microphone switch is pressed.

Your correspondent must appreciate this fact as this one-way-at-a-time conversation requires their co-operation. Be sure to warn all your possible correspondents about this beforehand as a lot of very expensive time can be wasted trying to explain the situation 'over the air'. It helps greatly if you can persuade them to say OVER when they have finished talking, too, even though they do not have a switch to press.

Procedure is much easier with a Duplex set as the set will automatically operate in the Duplex mode when switched to a two-frequency channel. Although the loudspeaker goes dead when the microphone switch is pressed, reception is retained in the earpiece (a telephone-type handset is always supplied with a Duplex set). Because of this, the microphone switch may be pressed and remain pressed for the duration of a normal telephone-type conversation on Duplex.

A Duplex set operates in the Simplex mode when switched to a single-frequency channel.

8.   When your correspondent replaces his or her handset (only *they* can stop the call, *you cannot*), a clock in the Coast Radio Station stops to record the time which forms the basis of the charge. *Do not* immediately switch back to Ch. 16 before the CRS Radio Officer has first advised you of the duration of the call.

There is a minimum charge of three minutes. For calls via Foreign Coast Radio Stations, the charge will be advised in French gold francs! Although French gold francs disappeared many years ago, along with gold sovereigns and guineas, this mythical currency is still used for international accountancy. Don't worry, though; British Telecom will sort it all out for you (for a small fee) and send a bill in pounds sterling to the name and address which was given in para. 3 of the Ship Radio Licence application. A table of current marine radiotelephone charges can be obtained from British Telecom (see the list of addresses at the back of the book).

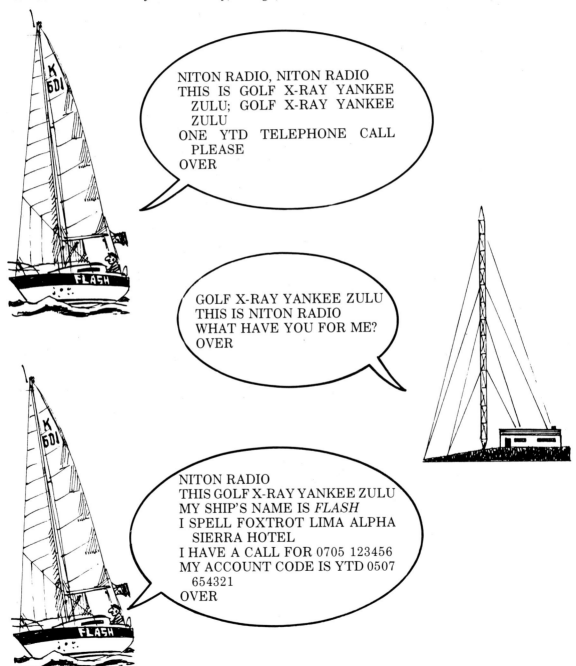

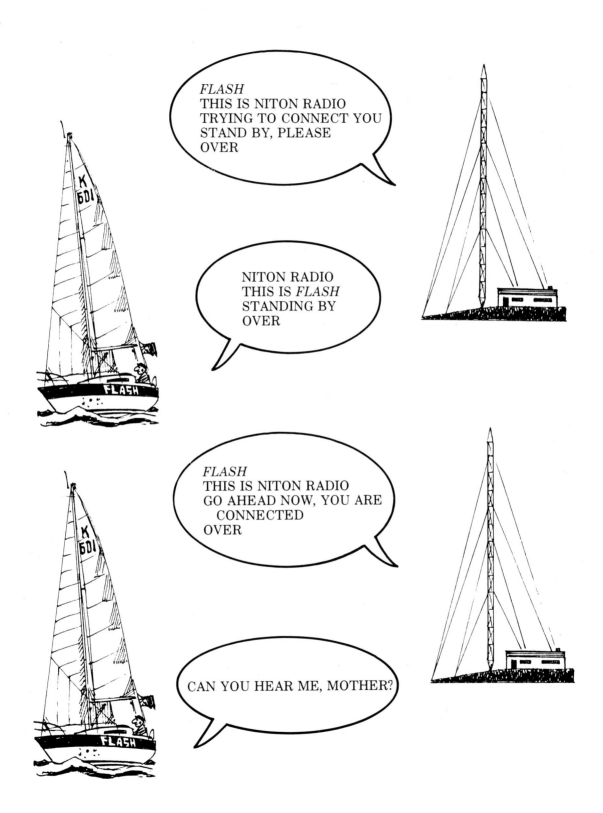

Telephone call via a Coast Radio Station

.... RADIO .... RADIO

THIS IS .... (call-sign)

.... (call-sign)

ONE (YTD) TELEPHONE CALL PLEASE

OVER

Coast Radio Station then replies, saying 'What have you for me, over'

.... RADIO

THIS IS .... (call-sign)

MY SHIP'S NAME IS ....

I SPELL ....

I HAVE A CALL FOR ....

MY ACCOUNTING CODE IS ⎰ YTD .... (UK only)

⎱ GOLF BRAVO ONE FOUR (non-UK)

OVER

DURATION OF CALL............... MINUTES.   CHARGE............... G.F.

A number of blank forms such as this could be kept on board near the radio set, with the ship's name, call-sign and accounting code filled in. Simply adding the other details for each call ensures fault-free procedure; the filled-in forms also act as a record of calls made.

Reversed charges

In addition to the 'YTD' and 'GB14' methods of direct payment, *transferred charge* ('reversed charge' or 'collect') calls can also be made. In this case, the recipient also pays an extra charge in addition to the cost of the call.

Radiotelephone log

Although there is no compulsion with voluntarily-equipped vessels, yachts are strongly advised to keep a reasonable record of transmissions made and important messages received (Q15). Officially called a 'Diary of the Radiotelephone Service', it should list:

● The operator's name with the date and times (GMT) at which he/she goes on and off watch.

● Times of departure from and arrival at ports, giving names of each.

● A summary of all communications relating to distress, urgency and safety.

● A record of communications between the vessel and shore stations or other vessels.

● Notes of important service incidents such as failures of power supply or breakdowns of apparatus.

● The position of the vessel at least once per day.

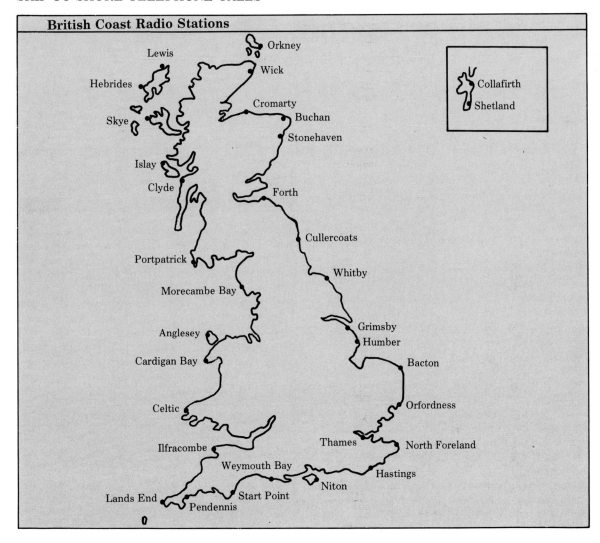

British Coast Radio Stations

Calls to ships from the shore

To call a ship using the ordinary telephone, dial Freephone, 0800-378389. This will be answered by 'Portishead Booking' as it is, actually, Portishead Radio at Burnham-on-Sea, Somerset. Although it operates only on the short wave band, Portishead Radio co-ordinates all Britain's shore-to-ship calls via Coast Radio Stations on MF and VHF as well as HF (short wave). The Radio Officer will ask for the ship's name and call-sign, approximate position or details of the voyage, name of the person called, the name and telephone number of the caller and how the call is to be charged. The caller will then be asked to 'ring off' and await re-call when the vessel has been contacted. There is a minimum charge of three minutes.

If the call is to a yacht, it is most likely that the radio will be operating in Simplex so be prepared to say 'OVER' to invite a reply after speaking!

Free Medical Advice

Coast Radio Stations can make free, untimed connections to doctors for medical advice at any time. Calls to British Coast Radio Stations *on their working channels* should be prefixed by PAN-PAN MEDICO spoken three times. The procedure with foreign stations is given in *ALRS*, Vol. 1.

In the case of known medical conditions (e.g. diving accidents) HM Coastguard can arrange MEDICAL ACTION (see p34).

11 Distress signal (Mayday)

To qualify for a distress signal, the situation must satisfy three important conditions (Q1).
- The *whole ship* must be in danger. So dismasting, heart attacks, man overboard, etc. do not qualify for MAYDAY.
- It must be *grave danger*, that is a threat to the lives of *everyone* on board. In other words a *disaster*.
- It must be *imminent danger*, that is not something which *may* happen in three or four hours' time but a disaster which is *certain* to happen during the next few minutes.

The precise circumstances of a situation can make all the difference between PAN-PAN and MAYDAY. For example; a motor yacht with engine failure ten miles south of Portland Bill, on a sunny afternoon in June in NW Force 3, is *not* in 'grave danger' although it certainly concerns the whole vessel and is certainly 'imminent' (in fact, it has just happened!). However, help may be required and the Coastguards should be alerted on Ch. 16 by preceding the call with PAN-PAN.

But the same situation, if it occurs 500 yards west of 'The Minkies' (Les Minquiers) on passage from Jersey to St Malo, in a NW Force 9, is certainly both grave *and* imminent!

Any decision to broadcast a MAYDAY signal (distress signals are always broadcast, that is not addressed to anyone in particular) or transmit a PAN-PAN call must be made by the master, that is the person in command of the vessel. The decision can be determined by the answer to this simple question: is my radio set about to disappear beneath the waves?

Answer yes: 'MAYDAY'

Answer no: 'PAN-PAN'

As the Mayday signal is a *broadcast* which could be received by people of all nationalities, there is a special sequence *which must be followed* if you are to be rescued quickly.
- First, the distress call to alert the world to your plight (Q2):

> MAYDAY, MAYDAY, MAYDAY,
> THIS IS (identity, identity, identity)

For identification purposes, either the vessel's name or call-sign may be used according to circumstances. If you start to sink in crowded waters and the vessel's name is emblazoned on the side in large, clear letters then that is your best identification. However, if no other vessel is close by and you are relying entirely on radio, the call-sign is the best identification.
- Second, the distress call is *immediately* followed (without waiting for an acknowledgement) by the *distress message* (Q2):

> MAYDAY (once again)
> IDENTITY (once again)
> MY POSITION IS . . . (Lat. and Long. *or* named spot *or* range and bearing *from* a well-known point of land)
> NATURE OF DISTRESS (e.g. 'SINKING', 'ON FIRE')
> ASSISTANCE REQUIRED (small boats actually sinking or on fire simply 'REQUEST IMMEDIATE ASSISTANCE' but, if drifting helplessly towards rocks could 'REQUEST TOW')
> NUMBER OF PEOPLE ON BOARD (don't distinguish between male/female, adult/child, captain/crew/passengers/kids-who-went-for-the-ride/babes-in-arms, etc. *Just count heads* including, of course, your own)
> ANY OTHER INFORMATION (to help people help you, you may be able to activate an EPIRB – Emergency Position Indicating Radio Beacon – or fire flares)
> OVER (even though you may be about to leap into a liferaft, leaving your R/T behind, the last word is always OVER!)

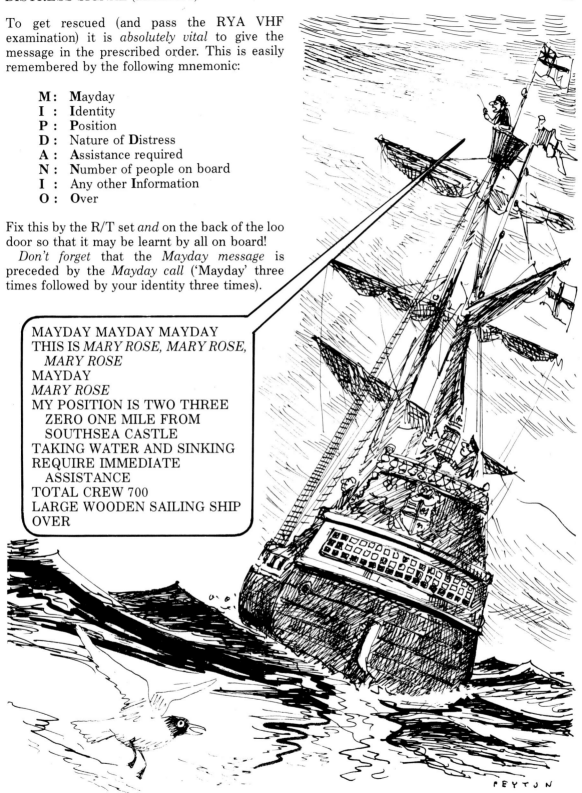

To get rescued (and pass the RYA VHF examination) it is *absolutely vital* to give the message in the prescribed order. This is easily remembered by the following mnemonic:

M : **M**ayday
I : **I**dentity
P : **P**osition
D : Nature of **D**istress
A : **A**ssistance required
N : **N**umber of people on board
I : Any other **I**nformation
O : **O**ver

Fix this by the R/T set *and* on the back of the loo door so that it may be learnt by all on board!

Don't forget that the *Mayday message* is preceded by the *Mayday call* ('Mayday' three times followed by your identity three times).

MAYDAY MAYDAY MAYDAY
THIS IS *MARY ROSE, MARY ROSE, MARY ROSE*
MAYDAY
MARY ROSE
MY POSITION IS TWO THREE ZERO ONE MILE FROM SOUTHSEA CASTLE
TAKING WATER AND SINKING
REQUIRE IMMEDIATE ASSISTANCE
TOTAL CREW 700
LARGE WOODEN SAILING SHIP
OVER

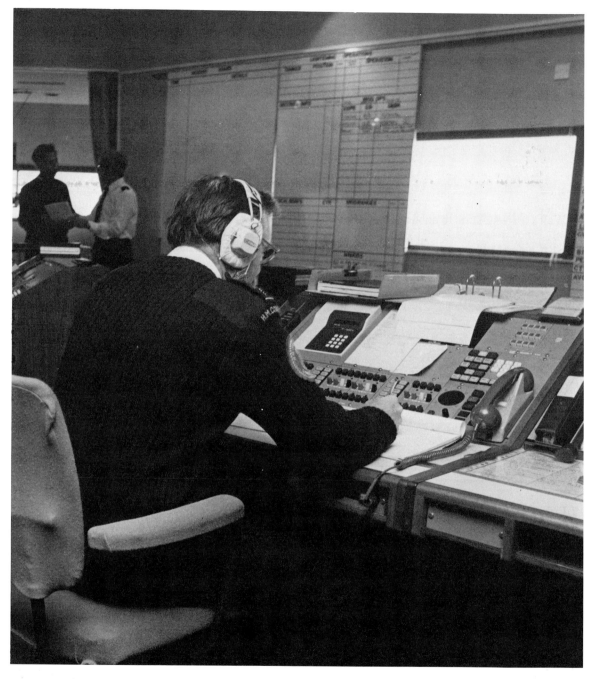

Above: The Operations Room at the Maritime Rescue Coordination Centre, Swansea.

12 Acknowledgement of distress signals

On hearing a distress signal (Q1)

● Listen and note the date, time and content of the message on the notepad with the pencil which is hung alongside the set – isn't it?
● Wait 10-15 seconds to ensure that the distress signal is not acknowledged by a Coastguard or Coast Radio Station.

If it is *not* acknowledged:

● Acknowledge receipt by saying:

> MAYDAY
> (Name or call-sign of distressed vessel
>   three times)
> THIS IS (your ship's name or call-sign
>   three times)
> RECEIVED
> MAYDAY

If you are able to offer practical assistance, add this information to your acknowledgement.

● Tell the world, by saying on Ch. 16:

> MAYDAY RELAY, MAYDAY
>   RELAY, MAYDAY RELAY
> THIS IS (identity), (identity), (identity)
> THE FOLLOWING DISTRESS
>   MESSAGE WAS RECEIVED
>   FROM (distressed vessel) AT (time)
> MESSAGE BEGINS . . . .
> MESSAGE ENDS
> OVER

If you hear the distress signal acknowledged by a Coastguard or Coast Radio Station and are able to offer assistance *call them* by preceding their name by the word MAYDAY. (All distress messages are preceded by the word MAYDAY).

If you hear the distress call acknowledged by a Coastguard or Coast Radio Station and are *not* able to render assistance, *keep quiet.*

On seeing a distress signal (Q1)

Broadcast the information by saying on Ch. 16:

> MAYDAY RELAY, MAYDAY
>   RELAY, MAYDAY RELAY
> THIS IS (your ship's name or call-sign
>   three times)
> MY POSITION IS (Lat. and Long. or
>   range and bearing *from* a well-known
>   point of land)
> (Type of distress signal seen)
> (Time distress signal was seen)
> (Position of distress signal seen *or*
>   bearing *from* your own position)
> OVER

Important procedural words (prowords)	
MAYDAY	Distress call for yourself (Q2)
MAYDAY RELAY	Distress call on behalf of someone else (Q1, Q3)
PAN-PAN	Indicates urgent call concerning the safety of a ship *or person* (e.g. man overboard) (Q12)
PAN-PAN MEDICO	Precedes a call to a *Coast Radio Station* requesting urgent medical advice. You will then be given a free telephone call to a doctor in the Accident Department of a local hospital (Q12) NOTE: French doctors speak only French! Most others speak English
SEELONCE MAYDAY	Radio silence on Ch. 16 is imposed by the station controlling distress communications using this phrase. Silence should be automatically observed during a distress situation (Q3)
SEELONCE DISTRESS	Radio silence on Ch. 16 imposed by any station other than the one controlling distress communications (Q3)
PRUDONCE	A concession, at the discretion of the controlling station, to allow essential signals on Ch. 16 – even though a distress situation may not be fully concluded (Q3)
SEELONCE FEENEE	End of radio silence (Q3)
SÉCURITÉ (SAY-CURE-EE-TAY)	Safety signal to indicate that a message of navigational importance is about to be sent (Q12)
SAY AGAIN	Repetition required (Q9)
ALL AFTER . . .	Everything following word or phrase indicated (Q9)
ALL BEFORE . . .	Everything prior to word or phrase indicated
ALL BETWEEN . . . AND . . .	Everything between words or phrases indicated
WORD AFTER, WORD WORD BEFORE, WORD BETWEEN	As above
STATION CALLING	(your ship's name or call-sign) Form of address to station which has called you but whose identification is in doubt (see below). If, on the other hand, you *think* someone is calling you, *do nothing*, but wait for the other station to repeat the call (Q6, Q9)
OVER	Invitation to other person to transmit (Q9)
OUT	End of conversation (Q9) NOTE: As the words OVER and OUT are contradictory it is *not* correct to end a transmission with OVER-AND-OUT! (Q9)
CORRECTION	The last word or phrase was wrong. This should be followed by I SAY AGAIN . . .
READ BACK	Repeat the message you have just received for confirmation that it was received correctly
RADIO CHECK	Tell me the strength and quality of my signal
I SPELL	I am about to spell the word just said in the International Phonetic Alphabet

Glossary

ALRS The *Admiralty List of Radio Signals*, the primary source of all information regarding radio stations, frequencies, etc. Available from Admiralty chart agents.

asl Above sea level (height of VHF aerials).

Authority to Operate on British Ships Normally granted when the radio operator passes the examination for the Certificate of Competence in Radiotelephony, but withheld from non-British candidates.

Call-sign Sequence of letters and/or figures allocated to a vessel equipped with a marine radiotelephone, e.g. GABC. Always spelt out phonetically over the air, it is less prone to misinterpretation than the vessel's name.

Capture effect On VHF, the radio locks on to the strongest signal and reproduces that to the exclusion of all others.

CB Citizens' Band radio; the unqualified 'free-for-all' band.

Certificate of Competence in Radiotelephony Granted to operators who have passed the appropriate examination, this is mandatory for all operators of marine radiotelephones.

Channel 16 The calling and Distress channel.

Channel M A private channel used by British marinas, yacht clubs, and British yachts which wish to communicate with them.

Coast Radio Station Shore-based 'telephone exchange' which links radio-equipped vessels with the international telephone system.

C.R.O.S.S.M.A. French coastguard service for the English Channel.

Dual Watch Electronic device fitted to marine VHF sets allowing two channels (Ch. 16 plus a selected channel) to be monitored at once.

Duplex Dual-frequency system allowing simultaneous two-way conversation by radio.

FM Frequency Modulation, the system by which signals are transmitted on the marine VHF band.

GB14 The Account Code of British Telecom, quoted by a British yacht when making a telephone call via a non-UK network.

International channels Marine VHF channels theoretically available to all marine VHF users, in practice restricted to certain well-defined uses.

MHz Megahertz, a measure of radio wave frequency in millions of cycles per second.

Private channel Channel allocated to a particular user and therefore not available for general use.

PTT switch Press-to-talk switch, employed on Simplex equipment to switch from receive to transmit mode.

Public correspondence channel Dual-frequency international channel employed for telephone system link-up; designed for Duplex operation but also available for Simplex-equipped stations.

Radio station Any radio-equipped building, ship or aircraft which has been allocated a call-sign.

R/T Radiotelephone.

Selcall Selective Calling system: a transmitted code which alerts a particular radio station.

Semi-Duplex Used in ship/shore correspondence when the Simplex equipment of the vessel makes Simplex procedure essential, despite 'Duplex' equipment of telephone user.

Ship's Wireless Licence Obligatory for all vessels equipped with marine R/T.

Simplex Single-frequency system allowing a radio station to receive *or* transmit, but not both at the same time.

Squelch Circuit employed in VHF radio sets to suppress background noise.

Traffic List List broadcast by Coast Radio Station to inform vessel that a correspondent wishes to make contact via the telephone system.

VHF Very High Frequency; the waveband used by the short-range marine radiotelephones fitted to yachts.

Working channel The channel on which business is transacted, following contact on Channel 16.

YTD Yacht Telephone Debit; the system by which the cost of a ship/shore telephone call is debited to the radio operator's own home telephone account.

Useful addresses

British Telecom International PLC
Maritime Radio
43 Bartholomew Close
London EC1A 7HP

Department of Trade & Industry
Radio Communications Division
Waterloo Bridge House
Waterloo Road
London SE1 8UA

Royal Yachting Association
RYA House, Romsey Road
Eastleigh
Hants SO5 4YA

Radio School Ltd
33 Island Close
Hayling Island
Hampshire PO11 0NJ

Examination centres

Southern
College of Maritime Studies
Warsash
Southampton
Hants

Isle of Wight
Club UK
Arctic Road
Cowes
Isle of Wight

Plymouth
Institute of Marine Studies
Plymouth Polytechnic
Drake Circus
Plymouth PL4 8AA

Falmouth
Falmouth Technical College
Killigrew Street, Falmouth
Cornwall

Bristol
Dept ACE, Brunel Technical College
Ashley Down, Bristol

London
City of London Polytechnic School of Navigation
100 The Minories, London EC3N 1JY

East Anglia
Lowestoft College of Further Education
Department of Marine Studies
St Peter Street, Lowestoft, Suffolk

Wales
South Glamorgan Institute of Higher Education
Department of Marine Studies
Western Avenue, Cardiff CF5 2YB

Yorkshire and Humberside
School of Engineering
Humberside College of Further Education
Queens Gardens, Hull HU1 3DH

Tyneside
South Tyneside College
Department of Nautical Science
St. George's Avenue
South Shields, Tyne & Wear NE34 6ET

Scotland
RYA Scotland, VHF Examinations
Caledonia House, South Gyle
Edinburgh EH12 9DQ

North West
Riversdale College of Technology
Department of Navigation, Riversdale Road
Liverpool Ll9 3QR

Northern Ireland
School of Maritime Studies, Ulster Polytechnic
Shore Road, Newtownabbey
Co. Antrim BT37 0QB

Jersey
VHF Radio Examinations, Highlands College
PO Box 142, Jersey, CI

Guernsey
College of Further Education
Route de Coutanchez
St Peter Port, Guernsey, CI

Examinations for servicemen are administered by Service sailing associations.